Vegan Keto Cookbook 2021:

Over 190 High-Fat Low-Carb Plant-Based Recipes to Shed Fat and Heal You from the Inside Out

Tyler MacDonald

© **Copyright 2021 by Tyler MacDonald - All rights reserved.**

The following Book is reproduced below with the goal of providing information that is as accurate and reliable as possible. Regardless, purchasing this Book can be seen as consent to the fact that both the publisher and the author of this book are in no way experts on the topics discussed within and that any recommendations or suggestions that are made herein are for entertainment purposes only. Professionals should be consulted as needed prior to undertaking any of the action endorsed herein.

This declaration is deemed fair and valid by both the American Bar Association and the Committee of Publishers Association and is legally binding throughout the United States.

Furthermore, the transmission, duplication, or reproduction of any of the following work including specific information will be considered an illegal act irrespective of if it is done electronically or in print. This extends to creating a secondary or tertiary copy of the work or a recorded copy and is only allowed with the expressed written consent from the Publisher. All additional rights reserved.

The information in the following pages is broadly considered a truthful and accurate account of facts and as such, any inattention, use, or misuse of the information in question by the reader will render any resulting actions solely under their purview. There are no scenarios in which the publisher or the original author of this work can be in any fashion deemed liable for any hardship or damages that may befall them after undertaking information described herein.

Additionally, the information in the following pages is intended only for informational purposes and should thus be thought of as universal. As befitting its nature, it is presented without assurance regarding its prolonged validity or interim quality. Trademarks that are mentioned are done without written consent and can in no way be considered an endorsement from the trademark holder.

Table of Contents

Introduction and Overview as a Keto Vegan 11
- Make Use of Low-Carb Substitutions 19
- Select Keto-Friendly Sweeteners 20
- Ketogenic Vegetable Choices 22
- Get Your Nutrients from Veggies 23
- Select Fresh Fruits 25

Chapter 1: Morning and Brunch Specialties 27

Begin a Ketogenic Routine 27
- Bulletproof Coffee 27
- Bulletproof Tea 29

Pancake Time 30
- Cinnamon Roll Pancakes 30
- Coconut Pancakes 32
- Crispy Flaxseed Waffles 33
- Flaxseed Pancakes 35
- Scallion Pancakes 36

Other Delicious Choices 38
- Almonds and Chips Breakfast Cereal 38
- Avocado – Carrot and Tahini Breakfast Bowl 39
- Bagel Thins for Breakfast 40
- Berry and Nut Cereal 42
- Blueberry Breakfast Cake – Flourless and Gluten-Free
  43
- Bran Muffins – Gluten-Free 45
- Breakfast Quiche 47
- Cinnamon Roll Muffins 48
- Macadamia Breakfast Bars 50
- Maple Walnut Breakfast Cereal 51
- Minty Eggplant Hash Browns 52
- Muesli in the Raw 53
- Peanut Butter Breakfast Cereal 54
- Psyllium Breakfast Mix 55

Pumpkin Pie Breakfast Cereal...56
Scrambled Tofu...57
Seed and Nut-Packed Bread 58
Vanilla and Turmeric Breakfast Cereal...........................60

Oatmeal and Porridge Favorites 61
Berries and Hemp Seeds 61
Blueberry Porridge...62
Fudge Oatmeal...64

Overnight Oat Options...65
Alternative #1: Vanilla Oats: The Base.............................65
Alternative #2: Pumpkin Spice Latte Overnight Oats.66
Alternative #3: Fudge Overnight Oats 67

Porridge Options...68
Delicious Plain Porridge..68
Porridge with Cinnamon and Hemp Hearts 69

Chapter 2: Delicious Meals and Salads.....................70

Meals..70
Asparagus and Mushrooms with Cauliflower Risotto .70
Asparagus and Tofu Stir Fry...73
Broccoli Noodles and Tofu 75
Cauliflower Tabbouleh 77
Collard Green Wraps..78
Crispy Tofu and Cauliflower Rice 79
Eggplant Lasagna 81
Falafel with Tahini Sauce 83
French Style Ratatouille 85
Green Panini..87
Sesame Tofu and Eggplant..88

Salads..90
Arugula and Blueberry Salad...90
Asian Zucchini Salad..91
Asparagus and Artichoke Salad...92
Avocado and Greens Salad...93
Avocado Papaya Salad..94
Bell Pepper and Asparagus Salad......................................95

Caesar Vegan Salad 96
Courgette Salad and Herbed Vinaigrette 97
Eggplant Salad 98
Kale Salad and Blueberry Dressing 99
Lemony Brussel Sprout Salad 101
Pear and Dates with Special Cider Dressing 102
Pecan Cauliflower Salad 103
Simple Green Salad with Lemon Vinaigrette 104
Sun-Dried Tomato Salad and Cider Dressing 106
Thai Peanut Zucchini Noodle Salad 107

Chapter 3: Healthy Soups – Stews and Chowder 109

Beetroot Ginger Soup 109
Broccoli and Cauliflower Soup 111
Cabbage and Beet Soup 112
Chili – Vegan Style 113
Chilled Minty Avocado Soup 114
Creamy Avocado Soup 115
Creamy Red Gazpacho Soup 116
Creamy Tomato Soup 118
Ginger Cauliflower Stew 120
Mushroom Soup 121
Red Onion Soup 123
Spanish Soup 124
Spinach and Turnip Soup 125
Superfood Keto Soup 126
Thai Pumpkin Soup 128
Turmeric Cabbage Soup 130
Zucchini Basil Soup 131

Chapter 4: Vegan Creams - Sauces and Dips 132

Avocado Mayo 132
Barbecue Sauce 133
Coconut Whipped Cream 134
Eggplant Bruschetta 135
Guacamole 136
Hummus and Avocado 137
Ketchup 138

Lemon and Jalapeno Cream Sauce 139
Mayo – Vegan Style 140
Nutella Spread 141
Peanut Sauce 142
Portobello Mushroom Bruschetta 143
Slow-Cooked Summer Bruschetta 144
Spinach Avocado Dip 145
Tahini and Cilantro Sauce 147
Tofu or Seitan Marinades 148
Vegan Sour Cream 151
Veggie Salsa 152

Chapter 5: Appetizers – Sides and Snacks 153

Sides *153*

Basil Zoodles and Olives 153
Beetroot and Pesto Noodles 154
Brussels Sprouts and Cashew Dip 155
Cabbage Slaw 156
Carrot and Zucchini Noodles in Thai Sauce 157
Cauliflower and Artichoke Couscous 158
Cauliflower Bites with Ranch Dip 159
Cherry Tomatoes and Zucchini Pasta 160
Chili and Coconut Cauliflower Rice 161
Coconut Cauliflower Rice 162
Creamy Curry Low-Carb Noodle Bowl 163
Edamame Kelp Noodles 165
Garlicky Mushrooms 166
Grilled Eggplant and Zucchini 167
Indian Curried Cauliflower 168
Kelp Noodles with Peanut Butter Sauce 169
Lime and Chili Carrot Noodles 170
Mediterranean Spaghetti Squash 171
Mushroom, Broccoli, and Squash Noodles 173
Nutty Pesto Zucchini 174
Pesto Kelp Noodles 175
Roasted Beetroot Noodles 176
Roasted Broccoli 177
Roasted Green Cabbage 179

- Roasted Kale and Squash 180
- Spaghetti Squash 181
- Sriracha Grilled Asparagus 182
- Teriyaki Grilled Eggplant 183
- Tofu Pizza Sticks 184
- Turnip Fries 185
- Turnip and Courgette Hash Browns 186
- Zucchini Noodles and Avocado Sauce 187

Snack Time Treats *188*
- Carrot Cake Bites 188
- Chocolate Granola 189
- Chocolate Protein Bars 190
- Cinnamon Granola 191
- Coconut and Peanut Butter Balls 192
- Fudge Balls 193
- Loaded Nut-Packed Coconut Granola 194
- Mushroom Chips 196
- Pecan and Maple Fat Bars 197
- Peanut Butter Fat Bombs 198
- Peanut Tofu Wrap 199
- Roasted Radish Chips 200
- Sweet Potato Toast 201
- Zucchini Chips 202

Chapter 6: Desserts – Smoothies and Beverages ... 203

Pudding Specialties *203*
- Avocado and Chocolate Pudding 203
- Chia Chocolate Pudding 205
- Chia Raspberry Pudding 207
- Chia Strawberry Pudding 208
- Coconut Chia and Turmeric Pudding 209
- Pumpkin and Peanut Butter Pudding 210

Other Delicious Desserts *211*
- Avocado Chocolate Mousse 211
- Banana Bread 213
- Cashew and Blueberry Cheesecake 214
- Chilled Avocado and Strawberry Bowl 215

Cinnamon and Pumpkin Fudge 216
Coconut Bombs..217
Coconut Cupcakes 218
Coconut Maple Fudge 220
Coconut and Peanut Butter Balls...............................221
Coconut and Strawberry Bars....................................222
Dairy-Free Chocolate Silk Pie....................................223
Lime Avocado Popsicles 225
Mexican Chocolate Avocado Ice Cream....................226
Minty Berries in A Dish 228
Pecan and Blueberry Crumble...................................229
Pumpkin Truffles.. 230
Raspberry Coconut Bark 231
Raspberry Truffles...232
Strawberry Ice Cream..233

Smoothies for Almost Any Occasion..............................*234*
Avocado Raspberry Smoothie 234
Banana Bread and Blueberry Smoothie 235
Berry Smoothie Bowl 236
Black Currant and Strawberry Smoothie 237
Blueberry Sensation 238
Chocolate and Mint Smoothie 239
Chocolate Smoothie 240
Cinnamon Chocolate Smoothie..................................241
Cinnamon Roll Smoothie 242
Easter Time Smoothie 243
Green Choco Smoothies 244
Maca Almond Smoothie 245
Minty Avocado and Spinach Smoothie 246
Pumpkin and Avocado Smoothie...............................247
Spinach and Cucumber Smoothie...............................248

Cold Beverages...*249*
Green Coffee Shake...249
Iced Blended Coffee 250
McKeto Strawberry Milkshake..................................251

Hot Beverages *252*
Coconut – Coffee Mug 252

  Creamy Hot Cocoa in the Crockpot 253
  Energizing Latte 254

A Final Word **255**
Keep Your Final Goals in Mind While on the Keto Journey
.... *260*
  More about those plateaus 263
  Benefits of Ketogenic Diet as a Vegan 264

Conclusion **267**
Index for the Recipes **269**

Introduction and Overview as a Keto Vegan

Congratulations on downloading *The Vegan Keto Cookbook 2021: Over 190 High-Fat Low-Carb Plant-Based Recipes to Shed and Heal You from the Inside Out.* By using the ketogenic diet with your vegan lifestyle, you are to receive many nutritional benefits from vegetables, fresh fruits, nuts, whole grains, and soy products among others.

These are some of those benefits along with the positive effects it brings to your body:

- **Antioxidants**
  With this addition, you can protect your body against several types of cancer.
- **Carbohydrates**
  Your body tends to burn your muscle tissue if you don't eat plenty of carbs.
- **Vitamin C**
  This works as an antioxidant and helps your bruises heal faster and keeps your gums healthy.
- **Protein**
  As a vegan, lentils, nuts, peas, and soy products provide this resource without health issues that can occur from red meats.
- **Fiber**
  The vegans experience better bowel movements with the increased high fiber in veggies and fruits.
- **Reduced Saturated Fats**
  Without the meats and dairy products, these levels lower immensely.

- **Magnesium**
  With the assistance of magnesium, calcium is better absorbed. It is found in dark leafy greens, seeds, and nuts.
- **Potassium**
  Acidity and water are balanced by potassium, which also leads to a reduction in cancer and cardiovascular diseases.

Some of the physical benefits can include body mass reduction, weight loss, higher energy levels, healthier skin, and many others. Supplements cannot replace a healthy diet plan, according to experts.

Walnuts are a known source for "brainpower" food, but also, the others mentioned below are considered as superfoods:

- **Almonds**
  You can help to regulate your blood pressure as well as having a good source as an energy booster. Its antioxidant qualities are loaded with fiber and calcium. Just ¼ of a cup of almonds provides eight grams of vegan protein.
- **Blueberries**
  The high content of flavonoid antioxidants is what is accountable to have shown enhancement in memory, as well as general cognitive function and learning. The flavonoid categories to stock up on include maqui, acai, and cacao.
- **Chia Seeds**
  The rich omega-3 fatty acid content is abundant in the chia seeds, which helps enhance memory and protect against cognitive decline. You also receive a lower calorie boost.
- **Pumpkin Seeds**
  Pumpkin seeds provide a boost of zinc, which enhances your thinking and memory skills. Have some in seasonal soups, by the handful, or in a hearty salad.
- **Cranberries**
  The high concentration of ursolic acid helps protect your brain cells from degeneration and injury, possibly even reversing the damage. Choose the sun-dried ones without sugar and use a bit of fruit juice for sweetener, or have some of the berries fresh, which is even more nutritious.
- **Strawberries**

Not only are these berries loaded with antioxidants, but they are also a good source of vitamin C, along with 21% RDA of manganese. Strawberries also help fight cancer.

You will also want to use special spices while on the ketogenic diet plan. Save some money and know what is in your spices. Use these in your unique dishes as a vegan. It's vital to read each of the spice labels since many spice manufacturers include sugar.

You can flavor your foods using these spices to remain in ketosis:

- **High-Quality Salts**
  While you're on the ketogenic diet plan, your insulin levels decrease. Your kidneys naturally excrete higher sodium levels, which in turn lower the potassium/sodium ratio in your body. Increase the amount of sodium with one of these choices:
  o Add 1/4 teaspoon of pink salt to your food or into a glass of water.
  o Have a bowl of vegan "bone" broth or use it in a keto recipe. (yes, you read that correctly...there is such a thing as vegan "bone" broth)
  o Have a snack of pumpkin seeds or macadamia nuts.
  o Add kelp or nori to your prepared foods.
  o Slice celery and cucumber – both have natural sodium content.

- **Cinnamon**
  Improve your insulin receptor activity by using cinnamon. Measure 1/2 teaspoon of cinnamon into a

of the keto recipes.

- **Homemade Pumpkin Pie Spice:** Use this simple low-carb concoction for a healthier pastry dish.

Pumpkin Pie Slice

Serving Yields: 10.75 tsp. – 1 tsp. per serving

Macros: 6.42 Calories| 0.8 g Net Carbs| 0.12 g Protein|0.09 g Total Fats

What You Need:
- Ground cinnamon – 2 tbsp.
- Ground nutmeg - .5 tsp.
- Ground ginger – 1 tbsp.
- Allspice - .5 tsp
- Cardamom - .25 tsp.
- Ground cloves - .5 tsp. or .75 tsp. whole cloves

How to Prepare:
1. Grind the cloves into powder using a spice grinder.
2. Combine all of the fixings in a mixing bowl until well combined
3. Store in a spice container to use any time the need arises.

- **Cayenne Pepper Hot Spices**

Sprinkling dishes with Cayenne pepper increases your metabolism, which helps burn away the fat. Cayenne is a stimulant for digestive enzymes and helps prevent stomach ulcers. Its anti-inflammatory elements make it a super choice for headaches, arthritis, or sore muscles. You can also receive a boost in your immunity as it clears away nasal congestion. Sprinkle your soups, stews, or chili.

- **Cumin Spice**
  This spice is an antioxidant and an excellent digestion reliever. It is a superior method to treat disorders such as bronchitis and asthma. It is also excellent for prediabetics or diabetes and also for removing body fat. It's a great source of vitamins A and C as well as iron.

- **Turmeric Spices**
  Dating back to Ayurveda and Chinese medicine, this Asian orange herb has been known for its anti-inflammatory elements. It is so easy to add to your delicious veggies and smoothies. These are some of its benefits
  - Excellent for weight management
  - Improves your digestion
  - Relieves arthritis
  - Helps control diabetes
  - Helps prevent Alzheimer's disease
  - Reduces your cholesterol levels
- **Spicy and Sweet Cloves**
  Add cloves to hot tea for a spicy change. The germicidal and antiseptic ingredients in cloves help ease many types of pain, including:
  - The smell of cloves can help encourage mental creativity
  - Relief of digestive problems
  - Fights infections
    - Helps relieve arthritis pain
    - Helps relieve gum and tooth pain

- **Clove Oil**
  Clove oil is beneficial as an antiseptic to kill bacteria in fungal infections, itchy rashes, bruises, or burns.

- **Basil**
  You can use either dried or fresh basil to maximize the benefits. Its dark green color indicates that it also maintains an outstanding source of calcium, magnesium, and vitamin K (good for your bones). Basil helps cure some of these conditions:
  - Inflammatory bowel conditions
  - Allergies
  - Arthritis

- **Star Anise**
  This is one spice that is commonly used in the United States and also is applied in Indian, Chinese, Indonesian, and Malaysian dishes. Its licorice-like taste pairs with tomatoes. It can be found in powder and "star" form purchased in the whole form. Simply substitute Chinese Five Spice, common anise, or fennel seed. It is a super choice for its antibacterial, antifungal, and antioxidant qualities.

  Other Useful Spices
  - Cilantro
  - Black Pepper
  - Chili Powder

- **Fermented Foods and Probiotics**
  Enjoy a dish of yogurt. You can also include items such as kimchee, sauerkraut, pickles, coconut milk, or water kefir to benefit your digestive system. Fermented foods help restore the "good" bacteria in your gut. The natural acids help stabilize your blood sugar levels as well as

the enzymes, probiotics, and other bioactive nutrients help support ketosis.

- **Healthy Fats**
  To achieve success in the ketogenic diet, you need fats. Fats are an essential part of your diet, but it is essential to know which ones are beneficial to your health and the ones that can be dangerous. Monounsaturated and Saturated Fats include avocado, coconut oil, and macadamia nuts are some of the recommended categories. These products can be incorporated into your meals using various recipes.

  Use non-hydrogenated lards or coconut oil. Less oxidation occurs in the oil because they have higher smoke points than other oils. These are some of those:

  - Avocado
  - Coconut Oil
  - Red Palm Oil
  - Sesame, avocado, and coconut oil
  - Flaxseed oil
  - Coconut flakes
  - Macadamia nuts
  - Macadamia Oil: One of the benefits of this oil is that it has a high smoke point. It carries a mild flavor, which is a super alternative to olive oil in mayonnaise.
  - Olives

- **Extra-Virgin Olive Oil (EVOO)**

Olive oil is one of the oldest edible oils in existence, with culinary uses dating back to at least 1000 B.C. and even more in the distance was the oil used for anointing priests and kings. It's versatile, delicious, and good for your health.

Research shows that olive oil helps prevent cardiovascular disease by protecting the integrity of your vascular system and lowering LDL "bad" cholesterol. Furthermore, after new research, extra-virgin olive oil also improves the gut microbiome by increasing the growth of probiotic Bifidobacterium strains.

Monounsaturated fats, like the ones in olive oil, are also linked with better blood sugar regulation, lower fasting glucose, and reducing inflammation throughout the body. Research further indicates that extra-virgin olive oil resists oxidation during the heating process much better than many other cooking oils, which makes it have a smoke point as high as 410°F.

Make Use of Low-Carb Substitutions

Chia Seeds
The seeds can absorb up to 11 times its weight in liquid. Be sure to add plenty of water and soak them for at least five minutes before using them in your keto recipes. Otherwise, you have some uncomfortable digestion after eating them. As always, be sure to remain hydrated.

Limes and Lemons
Your blood sugar levels naturally drop with these citric additions and also signal a boost in your liver function. Use them with a salad, in green juices, or cooked with meats or veggies. The following are the benefits of lime and lemon:

- Excellent for weight loss
- Balances pH
- Blood purifier

- Relieves respiratory infections
- Reduces fever
- Reduces toothache pain
- Boosts your immune system
- Decreases wrinkles and blemishes
- Flushes out the unwanted, unhealthy materials

Apple Cider Vinegar
You can add just one to two tablespoons of vinegar to an 8-ounce glass of water to help the process, or take a shot of vinegar solo. These are just a few ways this helps your progress:

- Helps you to drop the pounds
- Helps with sore muscles
- Improves your digestion tract
- Excellent for detoxification
- A good energy booster
- Reduces cholesterol
- Controls sugar intake/aids in diabetes
- Strengthens your immune system
- Balances your inner body system and functions

Select Keto-Friendly Sweeteners

Stevia Drops
Stevia Drops offer delicious flavors, including hazelnut, vanilla, English toffee, and chocolate. Enjoy making a satisfying cup of sweetened coffee or other healthy drinks. Some individuals think the drops are too bitter, so use only three drops to equal one teaspoon of sugar.

Pyure's Organic All-Purpose Blend
Pyure's Organic All-Purpose Blend is considered the best all-around sweetener with less of a bitter after-taste versus a stevia-based product. The blend of stevia and erythritol is an excellent alternative to baking, sweetening desserts, and various cooking needs.

The substitution ratio is one teaspoon of sugar for each one-third teaspoon of Pyure. Just add the blend slowly and adjust to your taste. You can always add a bit more. If you need powdered sugar, grind the sweetener in a NutriBullet or high-speed blender until it maintains a dry consistency.

Xylitol
This is excellent for sweetening your barbecue sauce and teriyaki; it tastes just like sugar! The naturally occurring sugar alcohol has the Glycemic index (GI) standing of 13. If you have tried others and weren't satisfied, this might be for you.

Xylitol also helps keep your mouth bacteria in check and is commonly found in chewing gum. However, don't use it often in large amounts since it can cause diarrhea - making chewing gum a laxative if used in large quantities.

Note: If you have a puppy in the house, be sure to use caution since it is toxic to dogs - even small amounts.

Swerve Granular Sweetener
Swerve is also an excellent choice as a blend. It's made of non-digestible carbs sourced from starchy root veggies and select fruits. Start with 3/4 of a teaspoon for every one of sugar. Increase the portion to your taste.

Swerve also has its own confectioner's powdered sugar for your baking needs. Unfortunately, it's more expensive (about twice the price) than other products such as the Pyure.

Pancake Syrup

Lakanto's Maple-Flavored Syrup is an exceptional choice for pancake syrup since it is "monk fruit" and erythritol-based.

Brown Sugar Option
Golden Monk Fruit Sweetener is an excellent choice for brown sugar. The name "monk fruit" came from the Buddhist monks over 1,000 years ago and is considered a cooling agent. It may not agree with your digestive system, so use it frugally if using in baked goods.

Ketogenic Vegetable Choices

Each of these has the Net Carbs listed per 100 grams or 1/2 cup:

- Alfalfa Seeds – Sprouted - 0.2
- Arugula – 2.05
- Asparagus – 1.78
- Bamboo shoots: 3.6
- Beet greens – 0.63
- Bell pepper
- Broccoli – 4.04
- Cabbage – Savoy – 3
- Carrots – 6.78
- Carrots – baby – 5.34
- Cauliflower – 2.97
- Celery – 1.37
- Chard – 2.14
- Chicory greens – 0.7
- Chives – 1.85
- Coriander – Cilantro Leaves – 0.87
- Cucumber with Peel – 3.13
- Eggplant – 2.88
- Garlic – 30.96
- Ginger root – 15.77
- Kale – 5.15
- Leeks – bulb (+) lower leaf – 12.35
- Lemongrass – citronella 25.31
- Lettuce – red leaf – 1.36
- Lettuce – crisp-head types ex. iceberg 1.77
- Mushrooms brown – 3.7
- Mustard Greens – 1.47
- Onions – yellow – 7.64
- Onions – scallions or spring – 4.74
- Onions – sweet – 6.65

Peppers – banana – 1.95
Peppers – red hot chili – 7.31
Peppers – jalapeno – 3.7
Peppers – sweet – green – 2.94
Peppers – sweet – red – 3.93
Peppers – sweet – yellow – 5.42
Portabella Mushrooms – 2.57
Pumpkin – 6
Radishes – 1.8
Seaweed – kelp – 8.27
Seaweed – spirulina - 2.02
Shiitake mushrooms – 4.29
Spinach – 1.43
Squash – crookneck - summer – 2.64
Squash - Zucchini – 2.11
Squash – winter – acorn – 8.92
Tomatoes – 2.69
Turnips – 4.63
Turnip Greens – 3.93
White Mushrooms – 2.26

You may want to consider these for your dieting needs as well:
- Parsnips
- Squash
- Peas
- Zucchini

Get Your Nutrients from Veggies

Calcium

Strong bones, muscle contraction, and proper blood clotting are all elements involved with calcium. Use these sources to add to your calcium counts:
- Leafy greens such as broccoli
- Dairy and non-dairy milk – unsweetened and zero carbs

You may need to supplement with calcium supplements, including Vitamin D, which is necessary for absorption. Both women and men should consume approximately 1000 mg — daily of calcium.

Vitamin D
Vitamin D supplies nutrients and hormones in your body. You cannot always get enough from your food, but you can go outside and take in some fresh air and sunshine for your portion. Use caution from over-exposure and the risks of skin cancer. The D vitamin also helps your body absorb magnesium, calcium, and other essential minerals to maintain your muscle growth and bone density. If yours is low, you are like about 1/3 of all Americans. Supplement the same by adding 400 IU per day as recommended, and add mushrooms to your diet plan.

Beta Carotene
Many foods contain beta carotene. However, a lot of them are higher in carbs, so the typically vegan keto dieter may not be getting a sufficient supply. Also, it should be noted that high levels of vitamin A in the body are toxic, so be careful if you are using supplements or try to get your beta carotene from whole food sources. Below is a list of several keto friendly foods that contain beta carotene:

- Asparagus
- Broccoli
- Collard Greens
- Dandelion Greens
- Kale
- Onions
- Peppers
- Spinach
- Pumpkin

Note: The brighter and more vibrant the yellow-orange color, the higher the levels of beta carotene; the chlorophyll hides the yellow-orange in leafy greens.

Chlorella
The green algae superfood is good for fighting off fatigue. It contains Chlorella Growth Factor – a nutrient containing DNA and RNA to help increase energy transport between your cells. You can purchase the supplement in powder form, tablets, or capsules. Mix it with water, a smoothie, or other drinks and have one daily.

Spirulina
The blue-green algae are similar to chlorella and contain all the amino acids your body requires, which makes it a complete protein. It also contains magnesium, iron, potassium, and other beneficial nutrients. It has superb antioxidant properties. The medication has shown positive results with individuals who suffer from cholesterol and high blood pressure. It raises the HDL (good cholesterol) and, at the same time, lowers the LDL (bad cholesterol). You can purchase in capsule form or in powder to mix in water or with a tasty smoothie.

Select Fresh Fruits

This collection of keto fruits for each 1/2 cup serving – listed in grams per serving:

- Apples – no skin - boiled – 13.6
- Apricots 7.5
- Bananas 23.4
- Blackberries – 23.1
- Blueberries – 22.1
- Cantaloupe - 6
- Kiwi – 14.2
- Oranges – 11.7
- Peaches – 11.6

- Pears – 19.2
- Pineapple – 11
- Plums – 16.3
- Kiwi - 15
- Watermelon 7.1

These are a few more that are acceptable for the Keto diet plan:

- Lemon juice
- Lime juice
- Strawberries
- Casaba Melon
- Green olives
- Avocados
- Coconut
- Rhubarb
- Black Olives
- Carambola aka Starfruit
- Gooseberries
- Acerola aka West Indian Cherry
- Oheloberries
- Boysenberries
- Grapefruit

Note: Values for the fruits and vegetables are rough estimates for general information. Each of the recipes using these items (in this book) has values calculated in the totals.

Let's see how all of these delicious recipes will blend with your chosen meals as you adjust to a new lifestyle. Please enjoy!

Chapter 1: Morning and Brunch Specialties

Begin a Ketogenic Routine

Start each morning (or your waking time) with a large glass of water. You can also add a supplement with MCT oil. Try this for maximum "get up and go" technique:

Bulletproof Coffee

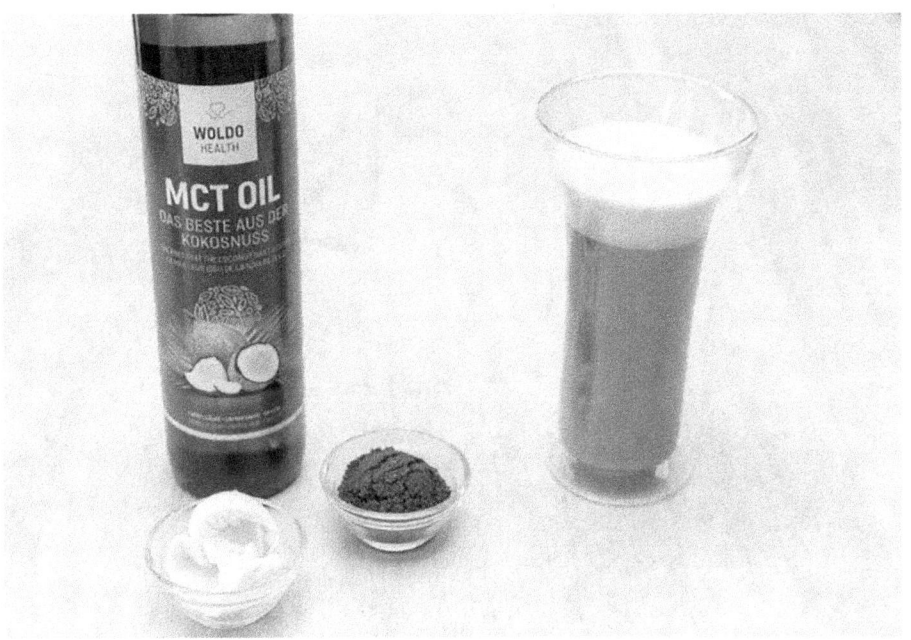

Nutritional Counts: Net Carbs: -0- g | Totals Fat: 51 g

Ingredients:
- MCT oil powder - 2 tbsp.

- Canned coconut milk - 2 tbsp.
- Hot coffee – 1.5 cups

Preparation Method:
1. Pour the hot coffee into your blender.
2. Add the powder and milk. Blend until creamy and frothy.
3. Enjoy served in a large mug at home or on-the-go.

Bulletproof Tea

Nutritional Counts: Net Carbs: 1 g| Total Fats: 17 g

Ingredients:
- Strong tea – 10 oz.
- Coconut or MCT oil – 1 tbsp.
- Canned coconut milk – 1 tbsp.
- Ground cinnamon - .125 tsp.
- Optional: Collagen peptides – 1 scoop

Preparation Method:
1. Combine all of the fixings in a tall mug.
2. Blend until frothy.

Pancake Time

Cinnamon Roll Pancakes

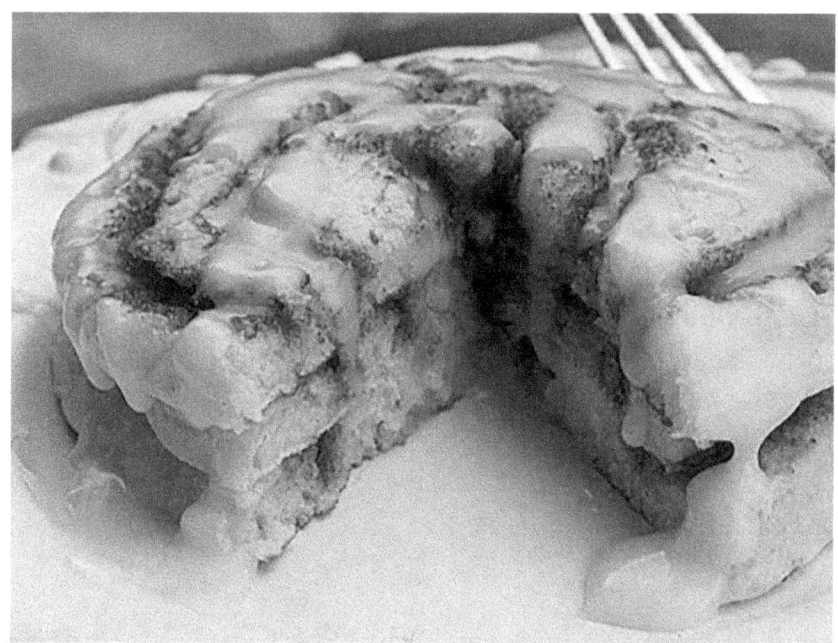

Serving Yields: 3
Nutritional Counts: Net Carbs: 0.5 g| Fat: 7 g

Ingredients:
- Rolled oats or quinoa flakes – 1 cup
- Milk of choice - .25 to .5 cup
- Unsweetened applesauce or sub. pumpkin - banana or sweet potato - .5 cup
- Cinnamon – 1 tsp.
- Apple cider vinegar or sub with lemon or lime juice – 1 tbsp.

- Baking powder – 1 tsp.
- Sticky sweetener of choice – 1 tbsp.
- Vanilla – 1 tsp.

For Cinnamon Roll Glaze:
- Coconut butter – 1-2 tbsp.
- Cinnamon – 1 tsp.
- Milk of choice – 1 tbsp.

Preparation Method:
1. In a high-speed blender, such as a NutriBullet, mix in each of your fixings and pulse until thoroughly combined and a thick batter remains.
2. Allow the batter to rest for 5-10 minutes, allowing the coconut flour/rolled oats to thicken. If it isn't thin enough, just continue adding milk a little at a time.
3. Preheat a greased/oiled pan over a low to medium temperature setting.
4. Pour scant 1/4 cup portions of batter on the hot pan. Cover the pan and cook for two to three minutes, until bubbles form on the edges. Then, just flip them over. Continue cooking until all the batter is used up.
5. Once pancakes are cooked, prepare your sticky cinnamon roll glaze. Melt your coconut butter and add the cinnamon. Thin out with milk and drizzle over the top.

Coconut Pancakes

Serving Yields: 2
Nutritional Counts: Net Carbs: 1 g| Fat: 7 g

Ingredients:
- Water – 1 cup
- Protein powder – 1 oz.
- Coconut flour - .25 cup
- Coconut oil - 1 tbsp.
- Baking powder – 1 tsp.
- Vanilla – 1 tsp.
- Psyllium husk powder – 2 tbsp. – to soak in .5 cup water

Preparation Method
1. In a mixing bowl, combine the dry components.
2. Combine the vanilla and coconut oil into the soaked psyllium husk.
3. Add water to the dry fixings, and mix it well.
4. Using the medium heat setting, spoon the batter into a warm skillet.
5. Cook for five minutes and flip. Continue cooking for 5 more minutes. Continue the process until you have your meal ready.
6. Serve and enjoy with your favorite toppings. Just be sure to add the extra carbs and fats.
7. Special Tip: The psyllium husk has many health benefits, including lowering your cholesterol and relieving constipation.

Crispy Flaxseed Waffles

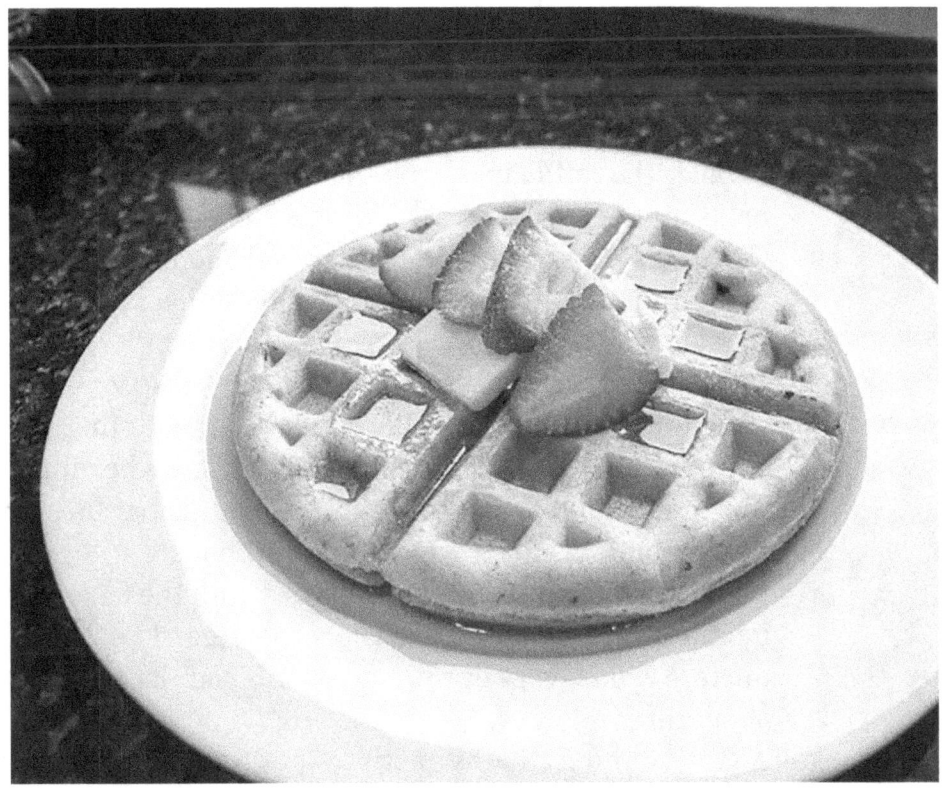

Serving Yields: 4
Nutritional Counts: Net Carbs: 3 g| Fat: 42 g

Ingredients:

- Roughly ground golden flaxseed – 2 cups
- Gluten-free baking powder – 1 tbsp.
- Sea salt – 1 tsp.
- Finely ground flaxseed – 5 tbsp. (+) 15 tbsp. warm water.
- Water - .5 cup

- Avocado oil or extra-virgin olive oil or melted coconut oil - .33 cup
- Fresh herbs – 1 tbsp. (if making savory) or 2 tsp. ground cinnamon

Preparation Method:
1. Arrange the waffle maker on the countertop and warm it up using the medium heat setting for crispy waffles.
2. Combine the sea salt with the flaxseed and baking powder in a big mixing container. Mix well and set to the side for now.
3. Pour the 15 tbsp. of warm water into the 5 tbsp. of ground flaxseed (replaces the regular egg) with the .5 cup of water. Let it sit for 5 minutes, and add the oil to the jug of a high-powered blender. Blend using the high setting until it is foamy or about 30 seconds.
4. Pour the liquid mixture into the bowl with the flaxseed mixture. Stir well until barely incorporated. The mixture will be very fluffy. Once combined, let it sit for about three minutes.
5. Add in your fresh herbs or stir in the ground cinnamon.
6. Divide mixture into 4 servings. Scoop each, one at a time, onto the preheated waffle maker and close the top. Cook until it beeps, and continue cooking with the remaining batter.
7. Eat immediately or freeze in an airtight container for a couple of weeks. It can be frozen and then toasted for a quick breakfast, lunch or dinner.
8. *Note:* You can also use 10 teaspoons of finely ground chia seed and 15 tablespoons of warm water (step 3). You can also garnish with some fresh strawberries.

Flaxseed Pancakes

Serving Yields: 1
Nutritional Counts: Net Carbs: 2.2 g| Fat: 27.1 g

Ingredients:
- Water - 3 tbsp.
- Flaxseeds – divided - 2 tbsp.
- Salt – 1 pinch
- Baking powder - .25 tsp.
- Coconut oil – 1.5 tbsp.
- Vanilla flavor vegan powder - .5 of a scoop

Preparation Method:
1. Combine the water with half (1 tbsp.) of the seeds. Stir in the oil. Set aside for a minute.
2. Whisk the baking powder, rest of the seeds, salt, and protein powder in a separate container.
3. Stir the fixings together and warm up a skillet (medium heat).
4. Add the batter to the prepared pan. Cook for five minutes on the first side. Gently turn the pancake and continue cooking for two more minutes. Do the same with the rest of the batter.

Scallion Pancakes

Serving Yields: 4
Nutritional Counts: Net Carbs: 4.7 g| Fat: 16.1 g

Ingredients:
- Scallions – white and green parts – sliced - 3
- Psyllium husk powder – 2 tbsp.
- Coconut flour - .5 cup
- Salt - .25 tsp.
- Garlic powder - .5 tsp.
- Sesame oil - .25 cup
- Warm water – 1 cup

Ingredients for the Sauce:
- Minced clove of garlic – 1
- Rice wine vinegar – 1 tsp.
- Water -1 tbsp.
- Sesame oil – 1 tsp.
- Tamari - 1 tbsp.
- Chili flakes – to taste

Preparation Method:
1. Mix the scallions, water, garlic, and salt in a container and set aside for about five minutes.
2. In another dish, whisk the husk powder and flour.
3. Combine the fixings to form a dough. Prepare into four portions and flatten using your hands.
4. Warm up the oil in a skillet. Place a dough round in the hot, flattening with the spatula. Cook for five minutes on each side and continue with the remainder of the dough sections.

5. Combine the sauce components and serve with the tasty scallion pancakes.

Other Delicious Choices

Almonds and Chips Breakfast Cereal

Serving Yields: 1
Nutritional Counts: Net Carbs: 3 g| Fat: 27 g

Ingredients:
- Coconut milk - .25 cup
- Hemp hearts – 3 tbsp.
- Shredded coconut - .5 tbsp.
- Chocolate chips - .5 tbsp.
- Chopped almonds - .5 tbsp.
- Liquid stevia – 1 drop

Preparation Method:
1. Combine the fixings in a jar or bowl with a lid.
2. Stir well and place in the fridge for a minimum of 4 hrs. (overnight is better).
3. Enjoy cold or warm.

Avocado – Carrot and Tahini Breakfast Bowl

Serving Yields: 1
Nutritional Counts: Net Carbs: 5.5 g| Fat: 52 g

Ingredients:
- Carrot - 1
- Haas avocado - 1
- Tahini – 2 tbsp.

For the SAUCE:
- Grated ginger – 1 tsp.
- Salt - .25 tsp.
- Lemon juice - .25 cup
- Olive oil - .25 cup
- Poppy seeds – 1 tbsp.

Preparation Method:
1. Slice the avocado in half and remove the pit. Shred the carrot. Set aside.
2. Whisk the sauce fixings. Mix the shredded carrot with 2 tbsp. of the sauce (save some for later).
3. Stuff the carrots into the avocado wells and sprinkle with the tahini.
4. Have a relaxing breakfast before you start your day.

Bagel Thins for Breakfast

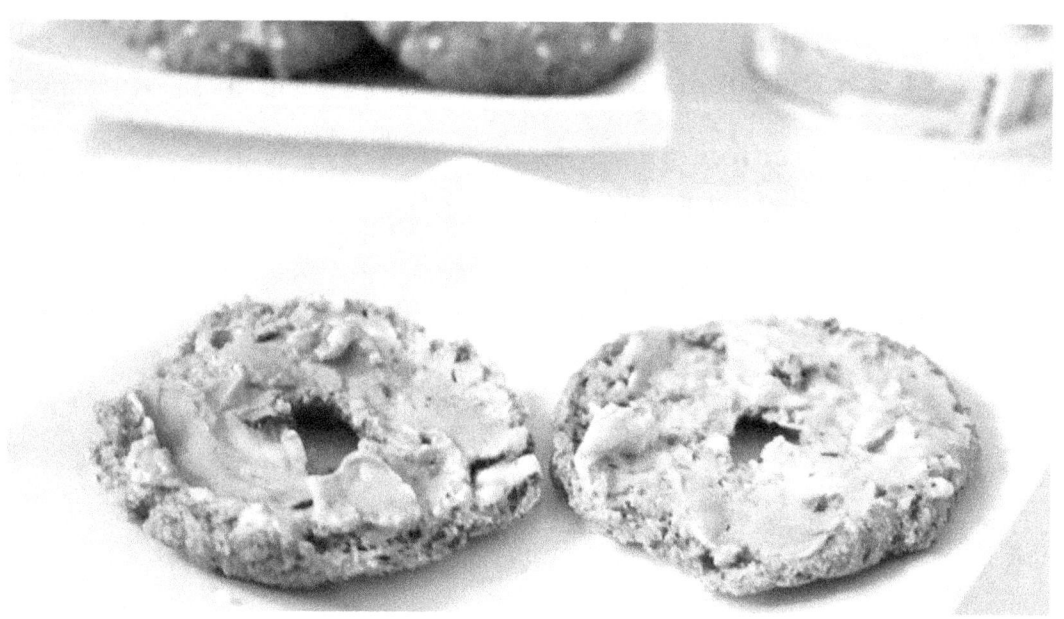

Serving Yields: 6
Nutritional Counts: Net Carbs: -0- g| Fat: 16.4 g

Ingredients:
- Ground flaxseed - .5 cup
- Tahini - .5 cup
- Psyllium husks - .25 cup
- Water – 1 cup
- Baking powder – 1 tsp.
- Salt – 1 pinch or add up to 1 tsp if using unsalted tahini)
- Optional - sesame seeds for garnish

Preparation Method:
1. Warm up the oven to 375°F.

2. Add the following to a mixing bowl: Psyllium husk, ground flax seeds, baking powder, and salt. Whisk until thoroughly combined. Pour in the water to the tahini, and whisk until combined.
3. Stir the dry ingredients into the wet, and then knead to form the dough. It's important that everything is kneaded thoroughly and that the dough is incorporated.
4. Form patties by hand that are about 4-inches in diameter and 1/4-inch thick. Lay on your baking tray and cut a small circle from the middle of each round.
5. You can also use a doughnut pan for this step, which makes everything so much easier!

Berry and Nut Cereal

Serving Yields: 1
Nutritional Counts: Net Carbs: 2.96 g| Fat: 32.59 g

Ingredients:
- Chopped strawberries - 2
- Blueberries - 2 tbsp.
- Walnuts - 2 tbsp.
- Pecans - 3 tbsp.
- Almonds - 3 tbsp.
- Sweetener to taste - 3 tbsp.
- For Serving: Coconut milk

Preparation Method:
1. Chop the almonds, pecans, and walnuts.
2. Combine each of the fixings into one mixing container (omit the milk).
3. Slowly add the milk last.

Blueberry Breakfast Cake – Flourless and Gluten-Free

Serving Yields: 12
Nutritional Counts: Net Carbs: 3 g| Fat: 11 g

Ingredients:
- Rolled oats - gluten-free ground into a flour – 2 cups
- Baking powder – 1 tbsp.
- Coconut palm sugar - .5 cup or any granulated sweetener of choice
- Sea salt – 1 pinch
- Milk of choice – 1 cup
- Flax egg – 1 (ground chia (+) 3 tbsp. water or 1 tbsp. of ground flax)
- Vanilla extract – 1 tsp.
- Smooth almond butter or any nut/seed butter of choice – 6 tbsp.
- Blueberries - .25 to .5 cup

Preparation Method:
1. Warm up the oven to reach 350°F.
2. Cover a square pan or loaf pan using a sheet of parchment paper and place to the side for now.
3. In a large container, add your dry fixings and stir well.
4. In another container, beat the eggs well. Stir in the melted coconut oil, unsweetened applesauce and sticky sweetener of choice and mix very well.
5. Mix each of the fixings in a high-speed blender until a smooth batter remains. Fold in the blueberries.
6. Pour your blueberry breakfast cake batter into the lined pan and bake for 35-40 minutes. Check for doneness

using a toothpick. It is done when it comes out clean from the center. Cool in the pan for about ten minutes.
7. Once the cake is cooled, prepare your frosting before topping the cake and cutting it into slices.

Bran Muffins – Gluten-Free

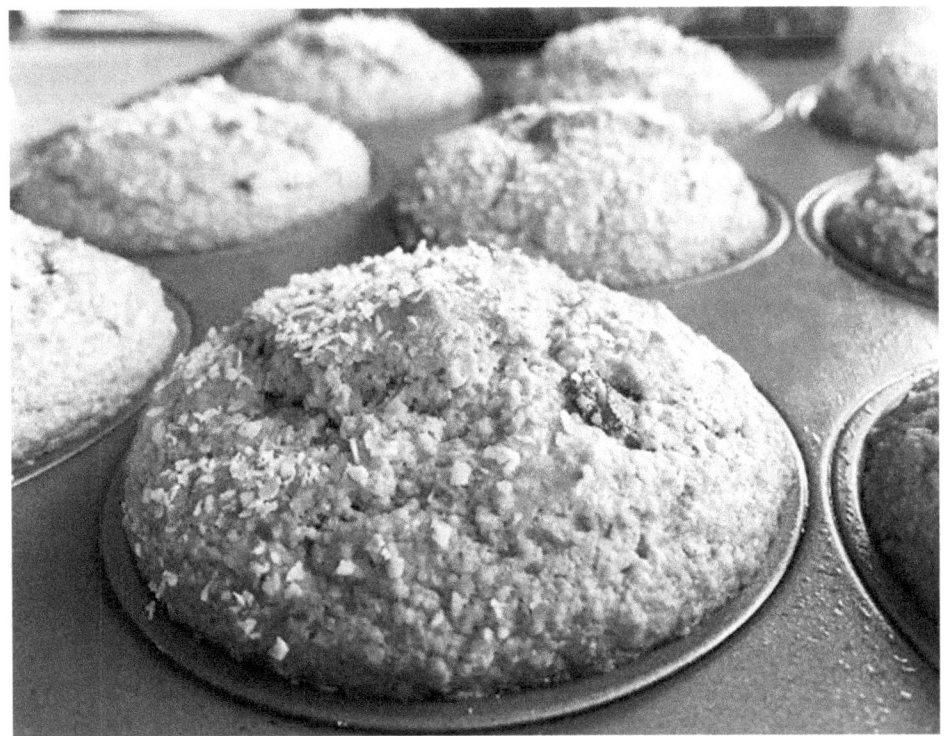

Serving Yields: 6
Nutritional Counts: Net Carbs: 1 g| Fat: 4 g

Ingredients:
- Ground flax - .5 cup
- Flax or chia eggs - 2
- Oat fiber - .25 cup
- Coconut flour – 2 tbsp.
- Baking soda - .25 tsp.
- Cinnamon - 1 tsp.
- Baking powder - .5 tsp
- Water - .25 cup

- <u>Lakanto Monk Fruit Sweetener</u> – or another granulated option - .5 cup or another granulated sweetener of choice
- <u>Vanilla extract</u> - .25 tsp.

Preparation Method:
1. Prepare the flax/chia eggs using 6 tbsp. of water and ground chia or 2 tbsp. of ground flax. Set aside.
2. Warm up the oven to reach 350°F. Spritz muffin tins with some non-stick cooking spray, and set aside.
3. Combine the oat fiber, 1/2 cup flax, sweetener, coconut flour, cinnamon, baking soda, and baking powder in a large mixing bowl. Mix well with a fork.
4. Pour in the water, vanilla extract, and flax/chia eggs. Mix well. Spoon into the prepared muffin tins.
5. Bake for 35 minutes.

Breakfast Quiche

Serving Yields: 5
Nutritional Counts: Net Carbs: 8.6 g| Fat: 37.7 g

Ingredients:
- Water – 3 tbsp.
- Olive oil – 2 tbsp.
- Chopped zucchini – 1.5 cups
- Salt - .5 tsp.
- Turmeric - .25 tsp.
- Black pepper – to taste
- Firm tofu – 14 oz.
- Low-carb vegan-friendly crust - 1

Preparation Method:
1. Program the oven setting to 350°F.
2. Warm up the oil in a skillet and slowly cook the zucchini.
3. Mix the turmeric, pepper, salt, tofu, and water until you reach a thick consistency.
4. Fold in the zucchini and stir well, adding the mixture to the crust.
5. Prepare for 30 minutes until the ingredients are set.
6. Relax and enjoy a slice of heaven!

Cinnamon Roll Muffins

Serving Yields: 20
Nutritional Counts: Net Carbs: -0- g| Fat: 9 g

Ingredients:
- Almond flour - .5 cup
- Vanilla protein powder 2 scoops (32-34 g per scoop)
- Baking powder – 1 tsp.
- Cinnamon – 1 tbsp.
- Nut or seed butter of choice almond, peanut, or sunflower seed butter, etc. - .5 cup
- Pumpkin puree can sub for unsweetened applesauce, mashed banana or mashed cooked sweet potato - .5 cup
- Coconut oil - .5 cup

for the glaze:
- Coconut butter - .25 cup
- Milk of choice - .25 cup
- Granulated sweetener of choice – 1 tbsp.
- Lemon juice – 2 tsp.

Preparation Method:
1. Heat up the oven temperature to reach 350°F.
2. Line a 12-count muffin tin with paper liners and set aside. This can also be made using a mini muffin tin.
3. In a large mixing container, mix your dry ingredients and mix well. Add your wet fixings. Combine well until fully incorporated.
4. Evenly distribute the cinnamon roll muffin batter evenly in the muffin liners.
5. Bake for 10-15 minutes, checking around the 10-minute mark by inserting a skewer in the center and seeing if it

comes out clean. If it does, muffins are done. Allow cooling in pan for 5 minutes, before transferring to a wire rack to cool completely.
6. Once cooled, prepare your cinnamon roll glaze by combining all ingredients and mixing until combined. Drizzle over the muffin tops and allow to firm up.
7. The muffins should be kept refrigerated for optimum freshness. They can be kept at room temperature, in a covered container, but must be eaten within 2 days. To freeze muffins, wrap each serving individually.

Macadamia Breakfast Bars

Serving Yields: 5
Nutritional Counts: Net Carbs: 9 g| Fat: 42 g

Ingredients:
- Coconut oil - .25 cup
- Crushed Macadamia nuts – 2.1 oz.
- Almond butter - .5 cup
- Unsweetened shredded coconut – 6 tbsp.
- Stevia drops - 20

Preparation Method:
1. Combine the fixings in a mixing container. Pour it into a parchment paper-lined baking dish.
2. Place in the refrigerator overnight for the best results.

Maple Walnut Breakfast Cereal

Serving Yields: 1
Nutritional Counts: Net Carbs: 2.47 g| Fat: 6.48 g

Ingredients:
- Chopped walnuts – 1 tbsp.
- Hemp hearts – 3 tbsp.
- Sugar-free maple syrup - .5 tbsp.
- Almond milk – 3 tbsp.
- Cinnamon - .5 tsp.
- Chia seeds – 1 tsp.

Preparation Method:
1. Combine the fixings in a jar or bowl.
2. Mix well and place in the fridge for at least four hours. Overnight is best.
3. Serve either cold or warm.

Minty Eggplant Hash Browns

Serving Yields: 8
Nutritional Counts: Net Carbs: 5.26 g| Fat: 6.4 g

Ingredients:
- Coconut oil – 2 tbsp.
- Red bell peppers - 2
- Eggplant - 1
- Garlic cloves - 4
- Red onion - 1
- Fresh mint leaves - .25 cup
- Toasted slivered almonds - .25 cup
- Sundried tomatoes in oil - .5 cup
- Ground cayenne pepper - .25 tsp.
- Ground coriander - .5 tsp.
- Ground cinnamon - .5 tsp.
- Salt and Pepper – to your liking

Preparation Method:
1. Prep the Veggies: Peel and cube the eggplant, mince the garlic cloves, and dice the peppers and onions.
2. Warm up the oil in a skillet. Sear the peppers and eggplant for 3 minutes – stir occasionally. Toss in the onion and garlic. Continue to saute for two additional minutes. Stir in the rest of the fixings.
3. Toss well and remove from the flame. Transfer to a serving platter and enjoy with your family and friends.

Muesli in the Raw

Serving Yields: 20
Nutritional Counts: Net Carbs: 4.2 g| Fat: 26 g

Ingredients:
- Unsweetened shredded coconut – 2 cups
- Ground linseed – 1 cup
- Sesame seeds – 1 cup
- Pumpkin seeds – 1 cup
- Pieces of walnuts – 1 cup
- Chopped almonds – 1 cup
- Sunflower seeds – 1 cup

Preparation Method:
1. Mix all of the fixings and seal in an airtight jar.
2. When ready to serve, just add some coconut cream and enjoy!
3. Note: Be sure to count the carbs for each serving to remain in ketosis.

Peanut Butter Breakfast Cereal

Serving Yields: 1
Nutrition Counts: Net Carbs: 3 g| Fat: 27 g

Ingredients:
- Hemp hearts – 3 tbsp.
- Peanut butter – 1 tbsp.
- Chia seeds – 1 tsp.
- Almond milk – 3 tbsp.
- Liquid stevia – 1 drop

Preparation Method:
1. Combine and mix the ingredients well in a bowl or mason jar.
2. Store the chosen container in the refrigerator overnight for the best results or for a minimum of four hours.
3. Serve hot or cold.

Psyllium Breakfast Mix

Serving Yields: 23
Nutritional Counts: Net Carbs: 2.3 g| Fat: 3.8 g

Ingredients:
- Hemp seeds – 7 tbsp.
- Ground flaxseed - 5 tbsp.
- Psyllium husk - 2 tbsp.
- Ground sesame - 2 tbsp.
- Dark unsweetened cocoa - 2 tbsp.
- Unsweetened coconut flakes - 5 tbsp.

Preparation Method:
1. Combine all of the components in a mason jar.
2. Seal the jar and shake well.
3. Serve with some black coffee or water.

Pumpkin Pie Breakfast Cereal

Serving Yields: 1
Nutritional Counts: Net Carbs: 3 g| Fat: 27 g

Ingredients:
- Pumpkin puree – 1 tbsp.
- Pumpkin pie spice - .5 tsp.
- Hemp hearts - 3 tbsp.
- Chia seeds – 1 tsp.
- Almond milk - 3 tbsp.
- Liquid stevia – 2 drops

Preparation Method:
1. Combine all of the fixings in a mason jar.
2. Mix well and refrigerate overnight for the best results.
3. Enjoy in the morning – either hot or cold.

Scrambled Tofu

Serving Yields: 4
Nutritional Counts: Net Carbs: 9.7 g| Fat: 11.5 g

Ingredients:
- Olive oil – 1 tbsp.
- Diced tomatoes - 1 can - 14.5 oz.
- Chopped green onions – 1 bunch
- Firm silken tofu - 1 pkg. - 12 oz.

Optional Fixings:
- Pepper and salt
- Ground turmeric
- Optional: Vegan cheese - .5 cup

Preparation Method:
1. Chop and saute the onions. Using medium heat, heat up oil in a skillet, and slowly cook the onions until translucent.
2. Blend in the tomatoes along with the juices and the mashed tofu.
3. Add the turmeric, pepper, and salt for flavoring and heat.
4. Garnish as desired.

Seed and Nut-Packed Bread

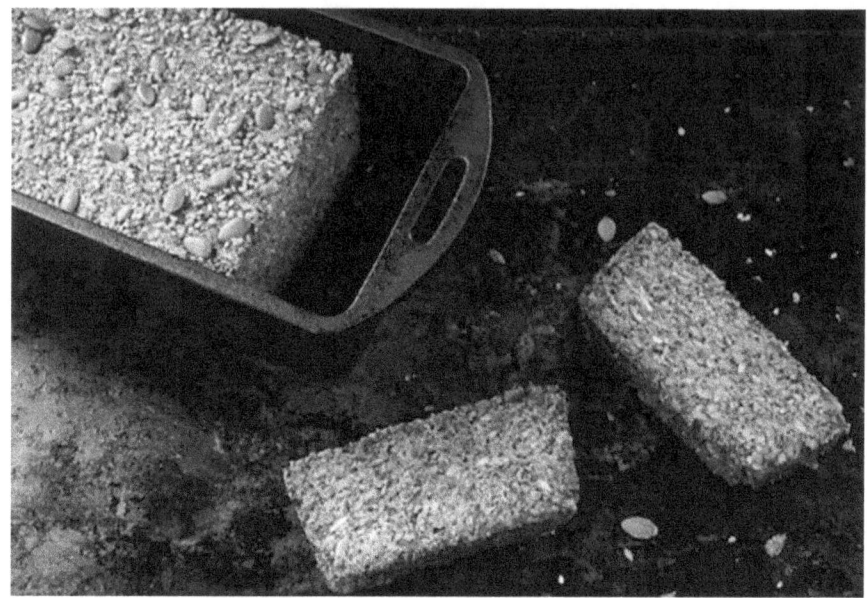

Serving Yields: 8
Nutritional Counts: Net Carbs: 4 g| Fat: 19 g

Ingredients:
- Psyllium husk powder – 3 tbsp.
- Sunflower seeds - .5 cup
- Pumpkin seeds - .5 cup
- Chia seeds – 2 tbsp.
- Onion powder – 1 tsp.
- Water - .33 cup
- Flaxseed meal - .33 cup
- Coconut oil - .33 cup
- Salt – 1 tsp.
- Almond slices - .33 cup

Preparation Method:
1. Prepare a baking tin with a sheet of parchment paper.
2. Warm up the oven to reach 350°F.
3. Combine the dry fixings in a mixing dish.
4. Stir in the oil until the mixture is crumbly.
5. Slowly add the water until it has the right dough consistency.
6. Spread it out in the pan. Arrange the pan in the preheated oven.
7. Bake for 15 minutes. Take it out and gently slice it into squares.
8. Put the pan back in the oven. Bake for 30 additional minutes.

Vanilla and Turmeric Breakfast Cereal

Serving Yields: 1
Nutritional Counts: Net Carbs: 3 g| Fat: 27 g

Ingredients:
- Coconut milk - .25 cup
- Chia seeds – 1 tsp.
- Hemp hearts – 3 tbsp.
- Liquid stevia – 2 drops
- Vanilla extract - .5 tsp.
- Turmeric powder - .5 tsp.

Preparation Method:
1. Mix together all of the fixings. Pour into a covered bowl or jar.
2. Refrigerate for at least four hours, but it's best if chilled overnight.
3. Serve either warm or cold.

Oatmeal and Porridge Favorites

Berries and Hemp Seeds

Serving Yields: 1
Nutritional Counts: Net Carbs: 3.10 g| Fat: 19.13 g

Ingredients:
- Boiling water - .5 cup
- Hemp hearts – 2 tbsp.
- Chia seeds – 1 tbsp.
- Unsweetened coconut flakes – 2 tbsp.
- For the Garnish: Stevia, cinnamon, and frozen berries – to your liking

Preparation Method:
1. Mix all of the fixings in a medium mixing container. Pour in the water. Stir well.
2. Let it steep for about 5 minutes and serve.

Blueberry Porridge

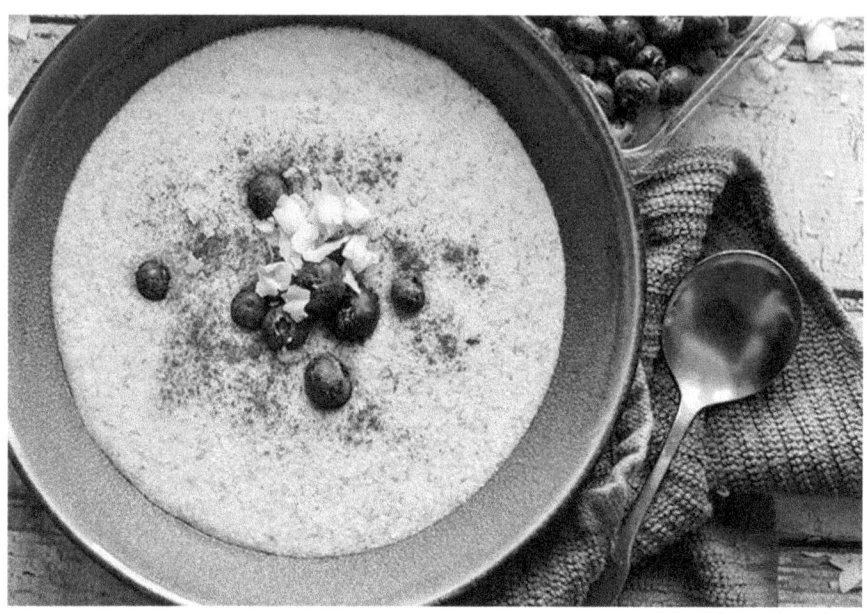

Serving Yields: 2
Nutritional Counts: Net Carbs: 8 g| Fat: 34 g

Ingredients:
- Almond milk – 1 cup
- Coconut flour - .25 cup
- Ground flaxseed - .25 cup
- Vanilla extract – 1 tsp.
- Cinnamon – 1 tsp.
- Liquid stevia – 10 drops
- Salt - 1 pinch

Preparation Method:

1. Warm up the milk on the stovetop using the low heat setting. Whisk in the cinnamon, salt, flaxseed, and flour.
2. At the time it begins bubbling, stir in the stevia and vanilla. Once it starts thickening, remove the porridge from the burner.
3. Serve and enjoy with a topping of blueberries, pumpkin seeds, and shaved coconut.

Fudge Oatmeal

Serving Yields: 2
Nutritional Counts: Net Carbs: 4.5 g| Fat: 39.4 g

Ingredients:
- Hemp hearts - .5 cup
- Full-fat coconut milk - .33 cup
- Sunflower butter - 1 tbsp.
- Chia seeds - 1 tbsp.
- Cacao powder – 2 tbsp.
- Liquid stevia – 3 drops
- Himalayan rock salt – finely ground – 1 pinch
- Vanilla extract - .5 tsp.

Preparation Method:
1. Mix all of the fixings in a mason jar and shake well.
2. Place in the fridge overnight for the tastiest results.

Overnight Oat Options

Alternative #1: Vanilla Oats: The Base

Serving Yields: 2
Nutritional Counts: Net Carbs: 2.9 g| Fat: 34.7 g

Ingredients:
- Full-fat coconut milk - .33 cup (+) more next day
- Hemp hearts - .5 cup
- Chia seeds – 1 tbsp.
- Liquid stevia – 3-4 drops
- Vanilla extract - .5 tsp.
- Himalayan rock salt – finely ground – A pinch

Ingredients for optional toppings:
- Whole raspberries - 6
- Whole almonds - 12

Preparation Method:
1. Combine all of the fixings into a container (12 oz. minimum) with a top.
2. Stir well and cover in the refrigerator 8 hours to overnight.
3. In the morning, add the milk if you like it and enjoy it.

Alternative #2: Pumpkin Spice Latte Overnight Oats

Serving Yields: 2
Nutritional Counts: Net Carbs: 9.4 g| Fat: 26.7 g

Ingredients:
- Canned pumpkin puree – 2 tbsp.
- Pumpkin spice or 3/8 tsp. –
    - Ground cinnamon - .5 tsp.
    - Ground cloves - .125 tsp.
    - Ground nutmeg - .25 tsp.
- 1 main recipe (Vanilla Oats: The Base: Variation 1)

Omit: 1/3 cup of the coconut milk and replace it with 1/3 cup of the brewed coffee.

Optional Toppings:
- Ground cinnamon
- Pecans

Alternative #3: Fudge Overnight Oats

Serving Yields: 2
Nutritional Counts: Net Carbs: 4.5 g| Fat: 39.4 g

Additional Ingredients:
- 1 recipe above (Vanilla Oats: The Base: Variation 1)
- Cacao powder – 2 tbsp.
- Sunflower butter – 1 tbsp.

Optional Toppings
- Cacao Nibs
- Shredded unsweetened coconut
- Strawberries

Porridge Options

Delicious Plain Porridge

Serving Yields: 1
Nutritional Counts: Net Carbs: 5.78 g |Fat: 13.1 g

Ingredients:
- Golden flaxseed meal – 3 tbsp.
- Coconut flour – 2 tbsp.
- Vanilla protein powder – vegan – 2 tbsp.
- Unsweetened almond milk – 1.5 cup
- Powdered erythritol – to your liking

Preparation Method:
1. Combine the flaxseed meal, flour, and protein powder in a bowl.
2. Pour the milk into a saucepan using the medium heat setting.
3. As the mixture thickens, stir in the sweetener (about .5 tbsp.).
4. Serve with your favorite garnishes but count those carbs.

Porridge with Cinnamon and Hemp Hearts

Serving Yields: 1
Nutritional Counts: Net Carbs: 3.6 g| Fat: 13.3 g

Ingredients:
- Freshly ground flaxseeds – 2 tbsp.
- Almond milk – unsweetened – 1 cup
- Alcohol-free stevia – 5 drops
- Chia seeds – 1 tbsp.
- Pure vanilla extract - .75 tsp.
- Hemp hearts - .5 cup
- Ground cinnamon - .5 tsp.

Ingredients for the toppings:
- Hemp hearts – 1 tbsp.
- Crushed almonds - .25 cup
- Brazil nuts - 3

Preparation Method:
1. Combine the fixings (omit the toppings for now) using a saucepan over medium heat.
2. Once the toppings are gently boiling, stir and continue cooking for another 2 minutes.
3. Take the pan from the burner and add the almonds and garnish with the hemp hearts and Brazil nuts.
4. Enjoy this yummy delight and prepare for your day!

Chapter 2: Delicious Meals and Salads

Meals

Asparagus and Mushrooms with Cauliflower Risotto

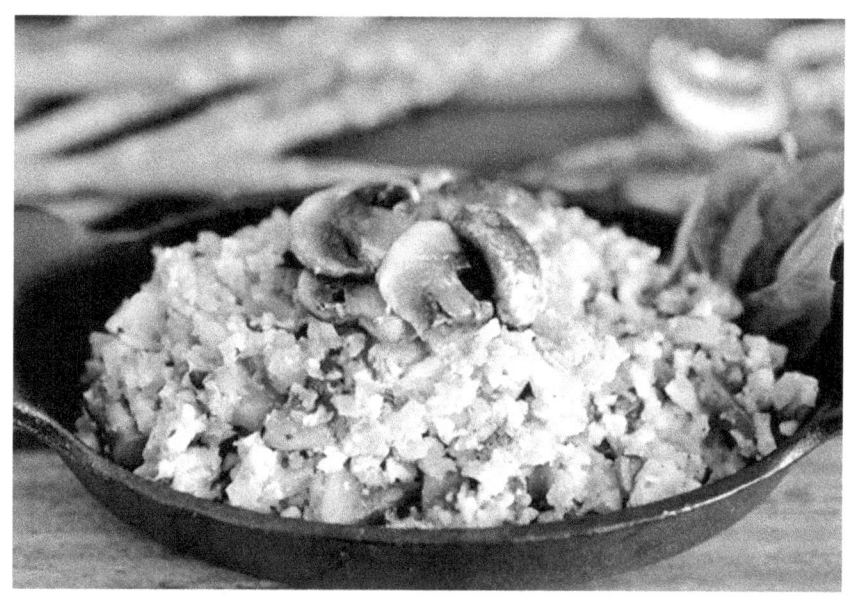

Serving Yields: 2
Nutritional Counts: Net Carbs: 9 g| Fat: 14 g

Ingredients:
- Large onion - .5 of 1
- Cauliflower rice – 7.5 oz.
- Garlic clove - 1
- Olive oil – 2 tbsp.

- Asparagus – 3 oz.
- Mushrooms – 4 oz.
- Lemon juice – 1 tbsp.
- White wine – 3 tbsp.
- Lemon zest - .5 of 1
- Parsley – finely chopped – 2 tbsp.

Preparation Method:
1. Prep the veggies by mincing the garlic and dicing the onions. Trim the asparagus into ½-inch pieces and slice the mushrooms.
2. Saute the garlic and onions in a hot skillet with the oil for 3-5 minutes. Toss in the mushrooms and continue cooking slowly for another minute.
3. Blend in the asparagus and cook for 2-3 minutes. Pour in the wine, lemon juice, and cauliflower rice.
4. Cook until tender for approximately 5-10 minutes.
5. Season to your liking and serve.

Asparagus and Tofu Stir Fry

Serving Yields: 3
Nutritional Counts: Net Carbs: 22 g| Fat: 24 g

Ingredients:
- Sliced extra-firm tofu – 8 oz.
- Ginger – peeled and grated – 1 tbsp.
- Sesame oil – 1-2 spritz
- Thinly sliced green onions - 4
- Toasted and chopped cashew nuts – 1 handful
- Tripped and chopped asparagus – 1 bunch
- Hoisin sauce – 2 tbsp.
- Basil -1 handful
- Mint - 1 handful
- Zest and juice – 1 lime
- Chopped spinach – 3 handfuls
- Salt – 1 pinch
- Chopped garlic cloves - 3

Preparation Method:
1. Prepare a wok with the oil and cook the tofu for a few minutes. Place on a platter.
2. Warm more oil and sauté the pepper flakes with the asparagus, onions, salt, and grated ginger. Cook for 1 minute.
3. Toss in the cashews, garlic, and spinach. Continue cooking for 1-2 minutes.
4. Add the tofu back in the mixture and add the lime juice, zest, and hoisin sauce.
5. Continue stir-frying for another 20 seconds.

6. Arrange on a serving platter and garnish with the mint and basil.

Broccoli Noodles and Tofu

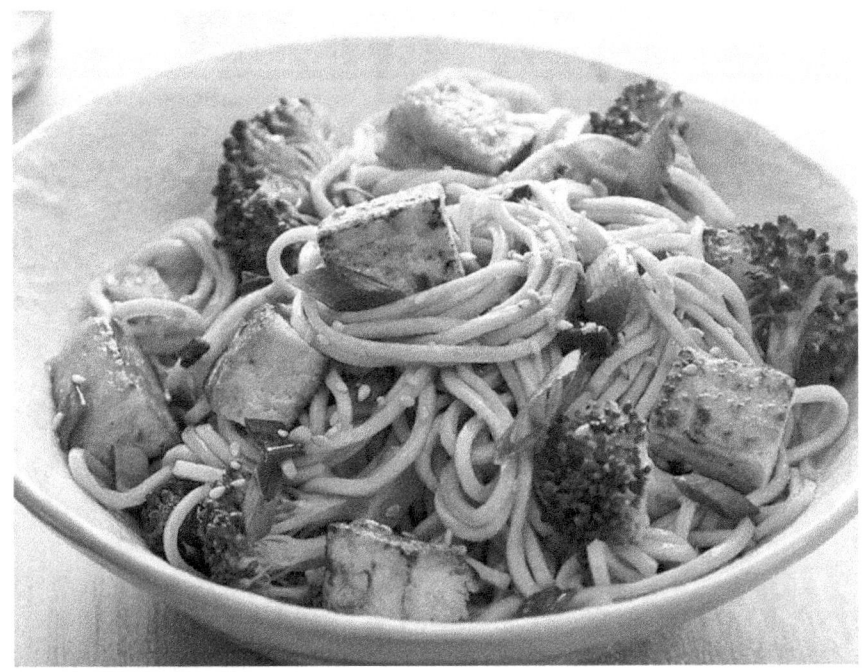

Serving Yields: 3
Nutritional Counts: Net Carbs: 14 g| Fat: 18 g

Ingredients:
- Broccoli stems – 2 spiralized
- EVOO – 2 tbsp.
- Diced onion - .5 of 1
- Extra-firm tofu - 1 block - 14 oz.
- Minced cloves of garlic - 2
- Finely diced red bell pepper - 1
- Cumin – 1 tsp.
- Turmeric – 1 tsp.
- Pepper and Salt – to taste

Preparation Method:
1. After a pot of water starts boiling, add the broccoli. Cook until done or about 2-3 minutes.
2. Warm up a pan with the oil. Once it is hot, start sautéing the onions, peppers, and garlic for three to four minutes. Stir in the cumin and cook for 1 minute.
3. Lastly, stir in the rest of the fixings and cook for two to three minutes.
4. Divide into three servings and enjoy.

Cauliflower Tabbouleh

Serving Yields: 8
Nutritional Counts: Net Carbs: 5.3 g| Fat: 7.19 g

Ingredients:
- Lightly steamed cauliflower rice – 2 cups
- Fresh mint – 1 cup
- Fresh parsley – 1 cup
- English cucumber - 1
- Red bell pepper - 1
- Cherry tomatoes - .5 lb.
- Red onion - 1
- EVOO - .25 cup
- Pepper and salt to taste
- Lemon juice - .25 cup

Preparation Method:
1. This is such a healthy treat. All it takes is adding the fixings into a bowl to toss.
2. Serve and enjoy anytime.

Collard Green Wraps

Serving Yields: 1
Nutritional Counts: Net Carbs: 3.1 g| Fat: 8.4 g

Ingredients:
- Sliced carrots - .25 cup
- Deveined collard greens - 2
- Sauerkraut - 2 tbsp.
- Tahini sauce - 2 tbsp.

Preparation Method:
1. Combine the sauerkraut and carrots and place inside the collard leaves.
2. Roll it into a wrap and drizzle with the sauce.

Crispy Tofu and Cauliflower Rice

Serving Yields: 2
Nutritional Counts: Net Carbs: 31.5 g| Fat: 34 g

Ingredients for the Stir-Fry:
- Toasted sesame oil – 1 tbsp.
- Extra-firm tofu - organic – 12 oz.
- Garlic cloves - 2 or 1 tbsp. minced
- Head cauliflower – 1 Small

Ingredients for the Sauce:
- Low-sodium soy sauce or tamari - .25 cup
- Toasted sesame oil- 1.5 tbsp.
- Light brown sugar – or another substitute - .25 cup
- Chili garlic sauce - .5 tsp.
- Natural almond butter - salted – 2.5 tbsp.

Optional Ingredients
- Veggies: Green onion, baby Bok choy, broccoli, red pepper, etc.
- *Suggested Toppings:* Cilantro, freshly squeezed lime juice, or sriracha

Preparation Method:
1. Drain the tofu about 1 1/2 hours before you plan to have dinner. Trim the bok down if it's larger than 12 ounces.
2. Roll the tofu in an absorbent towel several times. Put a heavy object on top to press it down. Place something like a cutting board with heavy canned goods or

similar objects; anything to add more weight. Do this for about 15 minutes.

3. Warm up the oven to 400°F and cube the tofu. Prepare a baking tin with a single sheet of parchment paper. Bake for 25 minutes until it has firmed up. When done, set it aside to cool.
4. Whisk the sauce fixings together until well mixed. Adjust the seasonings to your liking. Try adding a little more peanut butter to taste. Marinate to saturate the tofu for about 15 minutes.
5. Meanwhile, <u>rice the cauliflower</u> using a food processor or large grater. Set it aside.

6. Smash the garlic and prep the vegetables. Use the medium-high temperature setting and add the veggies. Cook them now in a dash of soy sauce and sesame oil. When done, cover them to keep warm.
7. Spoon the tofu into the preheated pan with several spoonfuls of the sauce to cover. Continue cooking until browned. When done, set aside.
8. Prepare the same skillet and spritz with some of the sesame oil. Toss in the riced cauliflower and garlic. Cover and steam the rice for about five to eight minutes or until tender and lightly browned and tender. Add more sauce and stir well.
9. Serve the rice topped with tofu and the prepared vegetables.

Eggplant Lasagna

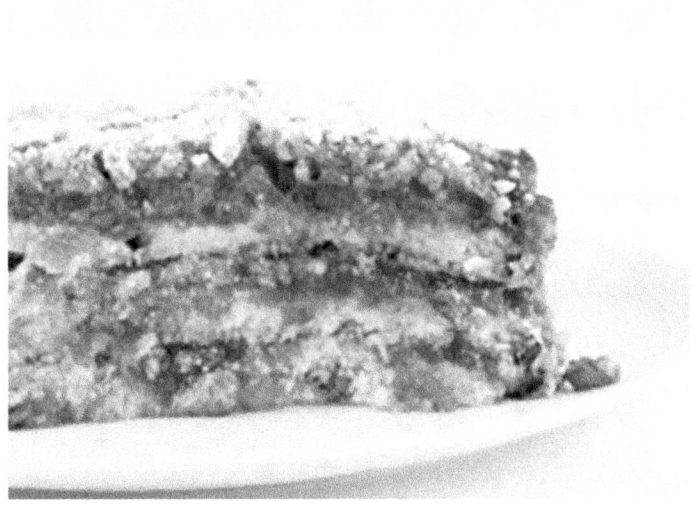

Serving Yields: 4
Nutritional Counts: Net Carbs: 4 g| Fat: 8 g

Ingredients:
- Sliced eggplant – 1
- Marinara sauce – 1 cup
- Salt – 1 tbsp.
- Vegan cheese of choice - .5 cup
- Vegan cashew ricotta – 1 cup
- Olive oil – as needed

Preparation Method:
1. Shake the salt over the eggplant rounds and set to the side for an hour. Rinse and pat them dry.
2. Lightly spritz a baking dish with the oil and layer the sliced eggplant on the bottom. Brush with the sauce and sprinkle with the cheese.

3. Add another layer of eggplant, ricotta, and lastly, the marinara sauce. Make one more layer of the eggplant, sauce, and cheese.
4. Bake with a lid on for 1/2 hour. Take the cover off and continue cooking for another 15 minutes before serving.

Falafel with Tahini Sauce

Serving Yields: 2
Nutritional Counts: Net Carbs: 5 g| Fat: 24 g

Ingredients:
- Raw pureed cauliflower – 1 cup or 1 med head - florets only
- Ground coriander - .5 tbsp.
- Ground cumin – 1 tbsp.
- Ground slivered almonds - .5 cup
- Kosher salt – 1 tsp.
- Minced garlic clove - 1
- Cayenne pepper - .5 tsp.
- Large eggs - 2
- Freshly chopped parsley – 2 tbsp.
- Coconut flour – 3 tbsp.

Ingredients for the Tahini Sauce:
- Water – 4 tbsp.
- Tahini paste – 2 tbsp.
- Salt – 1 tsp.
- Minced garlic clove -
- Lemon juice – 1 tbsp.
- For Cooking: Olive or grapeseed oil

Preparation Method:
1. Use a food processor and puree enough cauliflower to make one cup with a grainy texture. Process the almonds the same way, but don't over grind. Combine the fixings in a mixing bowl and add the remainder of the components of the recipe until well blended.

2. Warm up a half mixture of olive and grape seed oil. Make (eight) three-inch patties and add to the pan.
3. Cook until browned and turn them over. Four minutes for each side should be sufficient. Add them to a platter to drain on some paper towels.
4. Mix all of the tahini fixings in a bowl, adding small portions of water a little at a time until it reaches the desired thickness.
5. Use the tahini sauce as a garnish with the tomato and parsley.

French Style Ratatouille

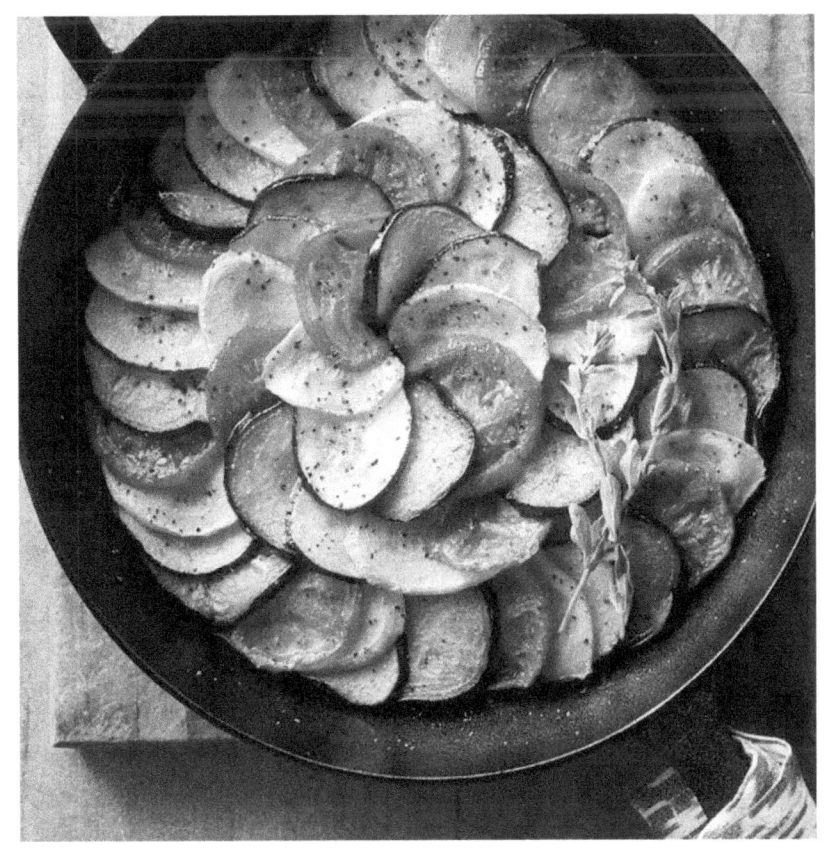

Serving Yields: 10
Nutritional Counts: Net Carbs: 9 g| Fat: 25 g

Ingredients:
- Eggplants – 2
- Tomatoes - 4
- Thyme sprigs - 4
- Zucchinis - 8
- Olive oil – 2 tbsp.

- Basil - .25 cup
- Garlic cloves - 3
- Yellow onions - 2
- Bell peppers - 3
- Salt – to your liking
- Bay leaf - 1

Preparation Method:
1. Prepare the veggies. Peel and cube the eggplant. Dice the onions and mince the cloves. Chop the rest of the vegetables.
2. Toss the eggplant with salt in a colander. Let it rest for a few minutes.
3. Warm up a Dutch oven with 1 teaspoon of oil. Sauté the onions for 10 minutes and add the salt. Add to the eggplant bowl. Rinse and squeeze all the water from the eggplant and cook for 10 minutes in the Dutch oven. Add to the veggie dish.
4. Warm up the rest of the oil and sauté the garlic. Add the tomatoes, thyme sprigs, and bay leaves.
5. Be sure to deglaze the bottom. Toss in the veggies and mix well.
6. Simmer and lower the heat setting for 45 minutes. Stir occasionally.
7. Trash the bay leaf and thyme when done and stir in the basil.
8. Serve for a very healthy meal for lunch or dinner.

Green Panini

Serving Yields: 1
Nutritional Counts: Net Carbs: 35.51 g| Fat: 55.21 g

Ingredients:
- Baby spinach – 1 cup
- Low-carb bread – 2 slices
- Pesto – 4 tbsp.
- Sliced avocado - .5 of 1
- Vegan butter – 1 tbsp.
- Pepper and salt – to your liking
- Hot sauce – 1-2 spritz

Preparation Method:
1. Use a knife to spread butter onto each slice of bread (only on one side). Spread pesto on the other side.
2. Add one slice in a skillet (low heat). Add some salt and pepper. Top it off with the avocado and spinach.
3. Add the slice of bread with the butter side facing out. Prepare until golden brown (3-4 min.). Flip and do the same.
4. Drizzle with the hot sauce and enjoy right away!

Sesame Tofu and Eggplant

Serving Yields: 4
Nutritional Counts: Net Carbs: 6.87 g| Fat: 24.45 g

Ingredients:
- Firm tofu block – 1 lb.
- Fresh cilantro - chopped – 1 cup
- Toasted sesame oil – 4 tbsp.
- Minced red pepper flakes – 1 tsp.
- Finely minced garlic– 2 cloves
- <u>Swerve confectioners</u> – 2 tsp.
- Eggplant -1 whole
- Unseasoned rice vinegar – 3 tbsp.
- Olive oil – 1 tbsp.
- To Taste – Salt and pepper
- Sesame seeds - .25 cup
- Soy sauce - .25 cup

Preparation Method:
1. Warm up the oven to 200°F. take the tofu block from the package and wrap it with a few paper towels
2. Place a heavy object such as a platter or cutting board with books or similar items on top. Let the water be pressed out.
3. Place the minced garlic, 2 tablespoons of sesame oil, cilantro, pepper flakes, rice vinegar, and sweetener into a large mixing bowl. Combine each of the components well.
4. Discard the peel from the eggplant. Julienne the eggplant with a mandolin with a julienne attachment –

for a uniform-looking noodle. Toss the marinade and eggplant together.
5. Pour the oil into a frying pan using the med-low temperature setting. Let the eggplant simmer until softened. You might need to add a little bit more oil, but remember to adjust the carbs or fats.
6. Turn off the oven and mix in the rest of the cilantro with the eggplant. Fold in the noodles to an oven-safe baking dish. Cover with a lid or a sheet of aluminum foil. Set it in the oven to keep warm.
7. Warm up the frying pan and slice the tofu into eight slices. Dip the tofu into some of the sesame seeds. Add two tbsp. of the sesame oil into the skillet. Fry both sides of the tofu for 5 seconds until they're crunchy.
8. Pour about 1/4 cup of soy sauce into the pan. Cover the pieces of tofu. Cook the slices until they appear browned and caramelized with the soy sauce.
9. Remove the noodles from the oven and plate the tofu on top.

Salads

Arugula and Blueberry Salad

Serving Yields: 6
Nutritional Counts: Net Carbs: 8 g| Fat: 10 g

Ingredients:
- Blueberries – 2 cups
- Arugula – 10 oz.
- Dijon mustard – 1 tbsp.
- Avocado oil - .25 cup
- Freshly squeezed orange juice – 2 tbsp.
- Balsamic vinegar – 2 tbsp.

Preparation Method:
1. Toss the arugula and berries into a salad dish.
2. Whisk the rest of the fixings in another cup.
3. Toss the dressing and salad together when it's time to eat.

Asian Zucchini Salad

Serving Yields: 10
Nutritional Counts: Net Carbs: 3.6 g| Fat: 9.3 g

Ingredients:
- Shredded cabbage – 1 lb.
- Thinly spiralized zucchini – 1
- Shelled sunflower seeds – 1 cup
- Sliced almonds – 1 cup
- Stevia drops – 1 tsp.
- Avocado oil - .75 cup
- White vinegar - .33 cup

Preparation Method:
1. Toss the cabbage, zucchini, sunflower seeds, and almonds in a salad dish.
2. Whisk the stevia, oil, and vinegar.
3. Toss the salad and drizzle with the delicious dressing.
4. Place in the refrigerator to get cold for about two hours before dinnertime.

Asparagus and Artichoke Salad

Serving Yields: 4
Nutritional Counts: Net Carbs: 7.93 g| Fat: 28.06 g

Ingredients:
- Artichoke hearts in oil – drain and wedge – 8
- Asparagus – 1 bunch
- Green beans - .5 lb.
- Capers – 1 tbsp.
- Freshly chopped oregano – 2 tsp.
- Toasted pine nuts - .25 cup
- Minced cloves of garlic – 2
- Olive oil - .25 cup
- Pepper and salt – as desired
- Lemon juice – 2 tbsp.

Preparation Method:
1. Chop the asparagus and green beans into strips. Drain and chop the capers and artichoke hearts.
2. Add a pinch of salt to a soup pot of water. Add the green beans and asparagus into the boiling water for 45 seconds. Drain in a mesh colander.
3. Add to a pot for an ice-water bath. Once they are chilled, just pat them dry with paper towels.
4. Toss all of the fixings into dishes and serve.

Avocado and Greens Salad

Serving Yields: 4
Nutritional Counts: Net Carbs: 7.8 g| Fat: 13.9 g

Ingredients:
- Mixed baby greens – 4 cups
- Sliced red onion – 1 tbsp.
- Sliced tomato – 1
- Peeled and sliced Haas avocado – 1
- Sliced cucumber – 1

Dressing Ingredients:
- Naval orange - .5 of 1
- Lime – 1
- Extra-virgin olive oil – 2 tbsp.
- A crushed clove of garlic – 1
- Oregano – 1 pinch
- To Taste: Freshly cracked pepper and salt

Preparation Method:
1. Toss all of the salad fixings into a salad dish or individuals bowls for a more accurate measurement.
2. Whisk the dressing ingredients well in another container.
3. When you are ready to eat, add the dressing, and enjoy!

Avocado Papaya Salad

Serving Yields: 6
Nutritional Counts: Net Carbs: 4.4 g| Fat: 8.4 g

Ingredients:
- Lime juice – 2 tbsp.
- Red onion – chopped – 2 tbsp.
- Diced Haas avocado – 2
- Chopped cilantro – 2 tbsp.
- To Taste – Pepper and Salt

Preparation Method:
1. Combine each of the fixings into individual dishes or one large one.
2. Serve when you're ready and enjoy.

Bell Pepper and Asparagus Salad

Serving Yields: 6
Nutritional Counts: Net Carbs: 5.1 g| Fat: 23.4 g

Ingredients:
- Sliced red onion – 1
- Sweet mini peppers – 17.5 oz.
- Freshly chopped asparagus – 14 oz.
- Apple cider vinegar – 3 tbsp.
- Extra-virgin olive oil - .5 cup
- Dijon mustard – 1 tbsp.
- Lemon – 1 zested
- Chopped bell pepper – 1 tsp.
- Finely chopped capers – 2 tbsp.
- Rosemary – 1 tbsp.
- Thyme – 1 tbsp.
- Himalayan salt – 1 tsp.
- Chopped walnuts - .5 cup

Preparation Method:
1. Thinly slice the mini peppers and dice the asparagus into small chunks. Slice the onion and finely chop the capers, rosemary, and thyme.
2. Combine all of the vegetables into a rimmed baking tin.
3. Whisk the rest of the fixings until thoroughly combined. Pour about 3/4 of the dressing into the veggies and toss.
4. Roast in the hot oven for 15 minutes.
5. Stir once or twice and broil for 5 to 6 minutes.

Caesar Vegan Salad

Serving Yields: 4
Nutritional Counts: Net Carbs: 5.2 g| Fat: 12.5 g

Ingredients:
- Ripe avocado - 1
- Lemon juice – 3 tbsp.
- Water – 2 tbsp.
- Garlic cloves - minced – 3
- Capers – 1 tbsp.
- Caper brine – 1 tbsp.
- Dijon mustard – 2 tsp.
- Hemp seeds - .25 cup
- Sea salt and fresh ground pepper, to taste
- Chopped romaine leaves – 12 cups

Preparation Method:
1. Add the lemon juice, avocado, water, garlic, capers, brine, mustard, salt and pepper to the blender or food processor. Blend until smooth.
2. You can add a little water if it's too thick. It will look similar to the consistency of pudding. Keep it this way to maintain the ultra-creaminess.
3. Spoon the dressing into a container and mix in the hemp seeds for that touch of parmesan similarity.
4. Arrange some of the lettuce in a large salad bowl. Spritz with the dressing and rotate the leaves to cover fully.
5. Serve immediately.

Courgette Salad and Herbed Vinaigrette

Serving Yields: 4
Nutritional Counts: Net Carbs: 1 g| Fat: 6 g

Ingredients:
- Olive oil – 2 tbsp.
- Lemon juiced – 1
- Chives- chopped - .5 of 1 pkg.
- Chopped mint - .5 of 1 pkg.
- Spiralized courgettes – 10.5 oz.
- To Your Liking: Pepper and salt

Preparation Method:
1. Use a spiralizer for the courgettes/zucchini.
2. Mix the oil with the pepper, salt, and lemon juice. Stir in the herbs.
3. Toss the noodles and dressing into a salad dish.
4. Toss and serve.

Eggplant Salad

Serving Yields: 6
Nutritional Counts: Net Carbs: 6 g| Fat: 9.4 g

Ingredients:
- Mashed cloves of garlic – 4
- Eggplants – 4
- Lemon juiced – 1
- Juiced white onion – 1
- Olive oil - .25 cup
- Chopped parsley – 1 handful
- Salt - .5 tsp.

Preparation Method:
1. Warm up the oven to reach 350°F.
2. Roast the eggplants for 45 minutes to one hour.
3. Whisk the parsley, garlic, olive oil, onion juice, and lemon juice. Together.
4. Scoop the flesh from the eggplants when done.
5. Combine the oil mixture with the salt. Stir well.

Kale Salad and Blueberry Dressing

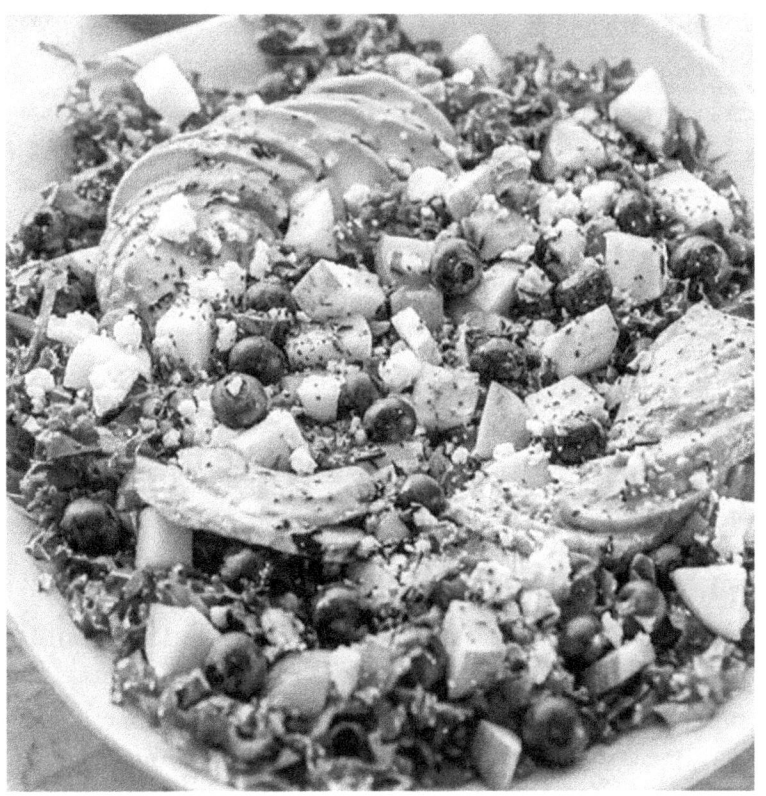

Serving Yields: 6
Nutritional Counts: Net Carbs: 10.5 g| Fat: 16 g

Ingredients:
- Freshly squeezed lime juice – 1 tbsp.
- Curly kale leaves – 6 cups – roughly torn
- Olive oil – 1 tsp.
- Ground black pepper - .5 tsp.
- Sea salt - .5 tsp.
- Avocado – 1
- Apple – 1

- Fresh blueberries - .25 cup
- Shelled and toasted pumpkin seeds – unsalted – 3 tbsp.
- Feta cheese from goat's milk - .25 cup - optional

Dressing Ingredients:
- Olive oil – 3 tbsp.
- Fresh blueberries - .25 cup
- Freshly minced ginger – 1 tsp.
- Raw honey – 1 tsp.
- Apple cider vinegar – 2 tbsp.
- Freshly cracked black pepper - .25 tsp.
- Sea salt - .25 tsp.
- Water – 3 tbsp.

Preparation Method:
1. Peel the apple and avocado. Remove the pit from the avocado. Dice both.
2. Combine the dressing fixings in a blender until creamy.
3. Combine the kale with the lime juice, pepper, salt, and oil. Use your hands and massage until wilted.
4. Arrange the kale on a serving dish and toss in the rest of the goodies.
5. Spritz with the salad dressing.

Lemony Brussel Sprout Salad

Serving Yields: 4
Nutritional Counts: Net Carbs: 2.5 g| Fat: 7 g

Ingredients:
- Brussel sprouts - 6 oz.
- Lemon – 1 – juiced
- Olive oil – 2 tbsp.
- Freshly ground black pepper and Kosher salt – as desired

Preparation Method:
1. Rinse the sprouts and trim away the ends. Slice them into halves and dice into fine bits.
2. Add sprouts to a salad platter and toss with the rest of the fixings.
3. Serve, smile, and enjoy.

Pear and Dates with Special Cider Dressing

Serving Yields: 4
Nutritional Counts: Net Carbs: 11.5 g| Fat: 25.6 g

Ingredients:
- Sliced fresh pear - .5 of 1
- Romaine lettuce – 2 cups
- Chopped and pitted Medjool dates – 2
- Walnuts – 1 handful
- Topping: Omega croutons

Dressing Ingredients:
- Olive oil - .25 cup
- Avocado – 1
- Ginger – 1 tbsp.
- Pitted Medjool dates - 2
- Water – 3 tbsp.
- Lemon juice – 2 tbsp.
- Dijon mustard- 1 tbsp.
- Herbamare - .25 tsp.

Preparation Method:
1. Combine all of the dressing fixings in the blender and combine until smooth.
2. Toss the salad components into salad dishes and add the dressing.
3. Add the croutons if using and serve.

Pecan Cauliflower Salad

Serving Yields: 8
Nutritional Counts: Net Carbs: 5.5 g| Fat: 9.2 g

Ingredients:
- Red and Yellow pepper - .5 cup of each
- Sliced thin purple cauliflower – 1
- Curly fresh kale – 4 cups – stem removed
- Chopped scallions - .5 cup
- Lemon juice – 1 cup
- Toasted – chopped pecans - .5 cup
- Olive oil – 3 tbsp.
- Pepper and salt to your liking

Preparation Method:
1. Chop the veggies and remove the stem from the kale.
2. Toss all of the fixings into a salad dish and serve.

Simple Green Salad with Lemon Vinaigrette

Serving Yields: 1

Ingredients for the dressing:
- Good quality olive oil or extra virgin oil - .25 cup
- Lemon juice – 3-4 cups
- Maple syrup – 1 tsp.
- Salt and black pepper – 1 pinch
- Optional: Minced shallot – 3 tbsp.

Ingredients for the salad:
- Organic mixed greens - 5 oz.
- Baby tomatoes - .25 cup
- Thinly sliced shallot or red onion - .25 cup
- Shredded carrots - .5 cup
- Optional: Pomegranate arils or dried fruit - .25 cup
- Salt and pepper - 1 pinch of each
- Toasted pepitas or sunflower seeds - 2 tbsp.

Preparation Method:
1. First, prepare the dressing by adding all of the fixings to a mixing bowl or into a small blender. Whisk or blend to thoroughly combine.
2. Taste and adjust the seasonings as needed by adding more maple syrup for sweetness, lemon for acidity, or salt or pepper to taste. Set aside.
3. Prepare the salad by adding the rinsed greens to a serving bowl or platter and topping with baby tomatoes, shallot or onion, carrots, pomegranate arils or dried fruit (optional), a pinch of salt and pepper, and toasted pepitas or sunflower seeds.

4. Add the dressing to the salad and toss to coat, or serve on the side. It's best when fresh.
5. Store salad separate from dressing if keeping for later use. Will keep in the refrigerator up to 2-3 days. Store the dressing in the refrigerator for 3-4 days. The oil can harden when cold, so let set out for a few minutes to warm and shake well to incorporate before serving leftovers.

Sun-Dried Tomato Salad and Cider Dressing

Serving Yields: 2
Nutritional Counts: Net Carbs: 11.3 g| Fat: 16.2 g

Ingredients:
- Chopped cucumber - .5 of 1
- Sun-dried tomatoes in the oil – 2 tbsp.
- Shaved carrots - 3
- Thinly sliced red pepper – 1
- Sunflower seeds – 1 tsp.

Dressing Ingredients:
- Dijon mustard – 1 tsp.
- Sunflower oil – 1 tsp.
- Apple cider vinegar – 1 tsp.
- Dried oregano - .25 tsp.
- Dried basil - .25 tsp.
- White powdered stevia – 1 pinch
- Herbamare - .125 tsp.

Preparation Method:
1. Toss all of the veggies into a salad mixing dish along with the sunflower seeds.
2. Whisk the dressing fixings well.
3. Pour the dressing over the tossed salad and serve.

Thai Peanut Zucchini Noodle Salad

Serving Yields: 4
Nutritional Counts: Net Carbs: 8 g| Fat: 12 g

Ingredients:
- Medium zucchini - 3 spiralized
- Carrot – 1 spiralized
- Chopped green onions - .25 cup
- Extra firm tofu, drained and cubed - .5 of 1 block
- Skinny Peanut Sauce - .5 cup (+) 1-2 tbsp. water
- Peanuts - .5 cup

for the SKINNY SAUCE:

Serving Yields: 18
Nutritional Counts: Net Carbs: 8 g| Fat: 12 g

Ingredients for the sauce:
- Protein Plus peanut flour - .25 cup
- Ginger – 1 tsp.
- Garlic powder - .5 tsp.
- Low-sodium soy sauce - gluten-free, if desired – 2 tbsp.
- Lakanto Liquid Monkfruit Sweetener or another liquid sweetener - 6 drops or to taste
- Lime juice - juice of 2 limes - 1 tbsp.
- Water - add more if desired – 2 tbsp.

Ingredients for the salad:
- Spiralized carrot- 1
- Medium spiralized zucchini - 3

- Diced green onions - .25 cup
- Extra-firm tofu - .5 of a block
- <u>Skinny Peanut Sauce</u>- .5 cup plus 1-2 Tbsp water
- Peanuts - .5 cup

Preparation Method:
1. Drain and cube the tofu. Prepare <u>the sauce</u> by adding the water until it's like you like it.
2. Combine the remainder of the fixings except for the peanuts in another container.
3. Top it off with the prepared salad dressing, and toss well. Sprinkle using some of the peanuts, and serve.

Chapter 3: Healthy Soups – Stews and Chowder

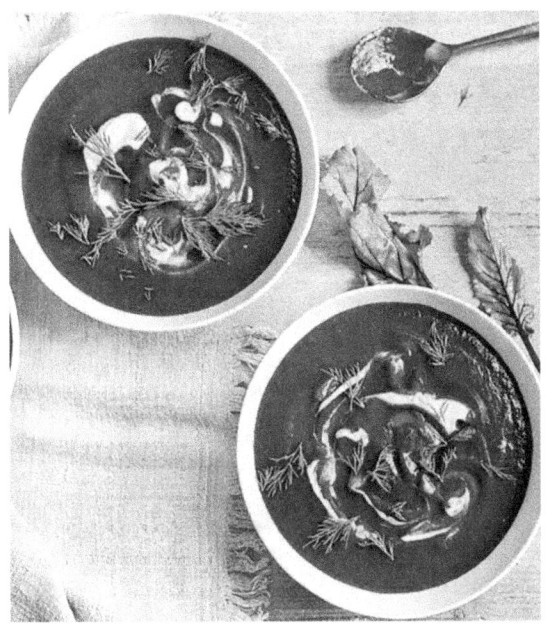

Beetroot Ginger Soup

Serving Yields: 2
Nutritional Counts: Net Carbs: 5 g| Fat: 12 g

Ingredients:
- Coconut milk - .5 of 1 can
- Chopped beetroots - 4
- Chopped onion – 1 peeled
- Fresh ginger - peeled and chopped – 3 tbsp.
- Black pepper and salt - .5 tsp. of ea.

- Coconut oil – 1 tbsp.
- Vegetable stock – 3 cups
- Garlic cloves - 3 minced

Preparation Method:
1. Warm up a saucepan and add the oil. Slowly cook the onion for 3-4 minutes.
2. Toss in the garlic and ginger. Sauté another 2 minutes.
3. Whisk the vegetable stock and beetroot together. Once it begins to simmer, just lower the heat. Simmer for about 20 minutes with a lid on the pot.
4. When done, remove from the burner and add the milk, pepper, and salt.
5. Make it creamy smooth with an immersion blender.

Broccoli and Cauliflower Soup

Serving Yields: 2
Nutritional Counts: Net Carbs: 6.1 g| Fat: 7.7 g

Ingredients:
- Cauliflower – 3.5 oz.
- Broccoli – 3.5 oz.
- Olive oil – 2 tsp.
- Chopped onion – 1 oz.
- Coconut milk - .25 cup
- White pepper and Pink salt – to your liking

Preparation Method:
1. Finely chop the broccoli and cauliflower.
2. Warm up a pan with the oil. Slowly add the onions and cook slowly until they are fragrant and translucent. Toss in the cauliflower, pepper, salt, and diluted coconut milk.
3. Pour in 1/2 of the broccoli and simmer 5-7 additional minutes. Let it cool a minute or so, and puree with an immersion blender.
4. Fold in the remainder of the broccoli.
5. Serve and enjoy!

Cabbage and Beet Soup

Serving Yields: 4
Nutritional Counts: Net Carbs: 6 g| Fat: 7 g

Ingredients:
- Shredded green cabbage – 2 cups
- Beets – 1 cup
- Carrots – 1 cup
- Olive oil – 2 tbsp.
- Vegetable stock – 3 cups
- Lemon juice – 1 tbsp.
- Garlic powder - .5 tsp.
- Onion powder - .5 tsp.
- Bay leaves - 2
- Juniper berries – 1 tbsp.
- Pepper and salt – to your liking

Preparation Method:
1. Shred the cabbage, beets, and carrots.
2. Warm up a saucepan with the oil. When it's hot, toss in the cabbage, carrots, and beets. Sauté 5 minutes.
3. Blend in the rest of the fixings and continue cooking until tender.
4. Strain out the juniper berries and bay leaves.
5. Let cool before serving.

Chili – Vegan Style

Serving Yields: 4
Nutritional Counts: Net Carbs: 2 g| Fat: 14 g

Ingredients:

- Green bell pepper - 1
- Red bell pepper – 1
- Textured vegetable protein – 2.5 oz.
- Soy sauce – keto-friendly – 1 tbsp.
- Vegetable oil – 1 tbsp.
- Diced canned tomatoes – 14 oz.
- Cooked black soybeans – 2 cups
- Minced cloves of garlic – 5
- Veggie broth - .5 cup
- Smoked paprika powder - .5 tsp.
- Oregano - .5 tsp.
- Chili powder - .5 tsp.

Preparation Method:
1. Dice the peppers and set aside.
2. Toss the vegetable protein into the saucepan and submerge it with water.
3. Warm up the oil in a pot. Sauté the peppers and textured vegetable protein for about five minutes. Whisk in the garlic and sauté for one minute. Stir in the rest of the fixings.
4. Once boiling, lower the heat and simmer for 10-15 minutes.
5. Serve.

Chilled Minty Avocado Soup

Serving Yields: 2
Nutritional Counts: Net Carbs: 4 g| Fat: 26 g

Ingredients:
- Romaine lettuce leaves - 2
- Ripe avocado - 1
- Lime juice – 1 tbsp.
- Chilled coconut milk – 1 cup
- Salt – to your liking
- Fresh mint leaves - 20

Preparation Method:
1. Add all of the fixings to a blender.
2. Mix well until creamy smooth.
3. Set aside for about ten minutes to cool.

Creamy Avocado Soup

Serving Yields: 4
Nutritional Counts: Net Carbs: 7 g| Fat: 31 g

Ingredients:
- Broccoli – florets – 1 head
- Minced garlic cloves - 2
- Chopped onion – 1
- Coconut oil – 2 tbsp.
- Vegetable stock – 1 cup
- Bay leaf - 1
- Coconut milk – 2 cups
- Pepper and salt – to your liking

Preparation Method:
1. Warm up a saucepan with the oil. When it's hot, add the onion and garlic. Sauté 5-6 minutes. Toss in the rest of the fixings.
2. Once it starts to boil, lower the heat setting and simmer for approximately 15-20 minutes. Trash the bay leaf.
3. Blend with an immersion blender and serve.

Creamy Red Gazpacho Soup

Serving Yields: 6
Nutritional Counts: Net Carbs: 8.5 g| Fat: 50.8 g

Ingredients:
- Medium tomatoes – 4-5
- Red peppers – 1 large
- Small green peppers – 2
- Medium avocados - 2
- Small red onion - 1
- Cloves of garlic - 2
- Fresh lemon juice - 2 tbsp.
- Wine vinegar/apple cider - 2 tbsp.
- Freshly chopped parsley - 2-4 tbsp.
- Medium spring onions – 2
- Freshly chopped basil - 2-4 tbsp.
- Large cucumber - 1
- Salt – such as Himalayan rock salt – 1 tsp.
- To your liking: Freshly cracked black pepper
- Feta cheese – 7.1 oz.
- EVOO – 1 cup
- Also needed: Parchment paper

Preparation Method:
1. Program the oven to 400°F.
2. Slice the peppers in half and deseed. Arrange them cut side down on parchment paper and roast them for approximately 20 minutes. The skin will turn black and blister.
3. Meanwhile, chop the red onion and add it to a pot. Cut up the tomatoes into quarter sections, and cut the avocado

in half and deseed, adding each to the pot with the onions.
4. Take the peppers out of the oven and cool. Throw away the skins and toss them into the pot. Blend in the garlic, fresh herbs, olive oil, pepper, salt, vinegar, and lemon juice. Pulse with a hand mixer until smooth. (Reserve a bit of the oil for garnishing.)
5. Dice the onion and cucumber, and add to the soup mixing well, seasoning to taste as desired.
6. Serve and top with some fresh herbs and a drizzle of olive oil (about 1 tablespoon for each serving).
7. *Note*: You can mix and match the types of peppers to change the coloring of the soup.

Creamy Tomato Soup

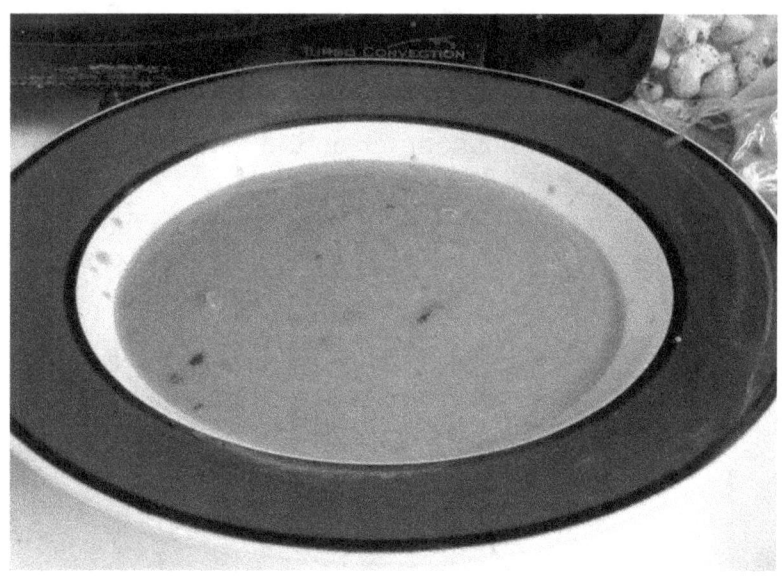

Serving Yields: 4
Nutritional Counts: Net Carbs: 7.7 g| Fat: 15.9 g

Ingredients:
- Sun-dried tomatoes - .5 cup
- Raw macadamia nuts - .5 cup
- Roma tomatoes - 4
- White pepper - .5 tsp.
- Sea salt – 1 tsp.
- Black pepper - .25 tsp.
- Garlic clove - 1
- Hot water – 4 cups
- Fresh basil - .25 cup

Preparation Method:

1. Toss each of the components into a high-speed blender.
2. Prepare for 5 minutes.
3. Serve in a warm bowl.

Ginger Cauliflower Stew

Serving Yields: 6
Nutritional Counts: Net Carbs: 12 g| Fat: 24 g

Ingredients:
- Tomatoes – 3
- Onion – 1
- Coconut oil – 2 tbsp.
- Cumin seeds – 1 tsp.
- Chopped kale – 1 cup
- Cauliflower florets – 1 head
- Jalapeno – seeded – 1
- Cumin powder – 1 tbsp.
- Ginger paste – 2 tsp.
- Turmeric powder – 1 tsp.
- Coriander powder – 1 tbsp.
- Coconut milk – full-fat unsweetened – 1 can
- Chopped cilantro – 2 tbsp.
- Sea salt – 1 tsp.

Preparation Method:
1. Finely chop the kale, jalapeno, tomatoes, and onions. Separate the cauliflower into florets.
2. Warm up the oil in a soup pot and toss in the cumin seeds. Sauté the onions for 1 minute and fold in the tomatoes. Simmer a minute or two and add the rest of the fixings.
3. Cover the pot and simmer for 15 minutes – making sure to stir after each 5-minute segment.
4. Serve and enjoy.

Mushroom Soup

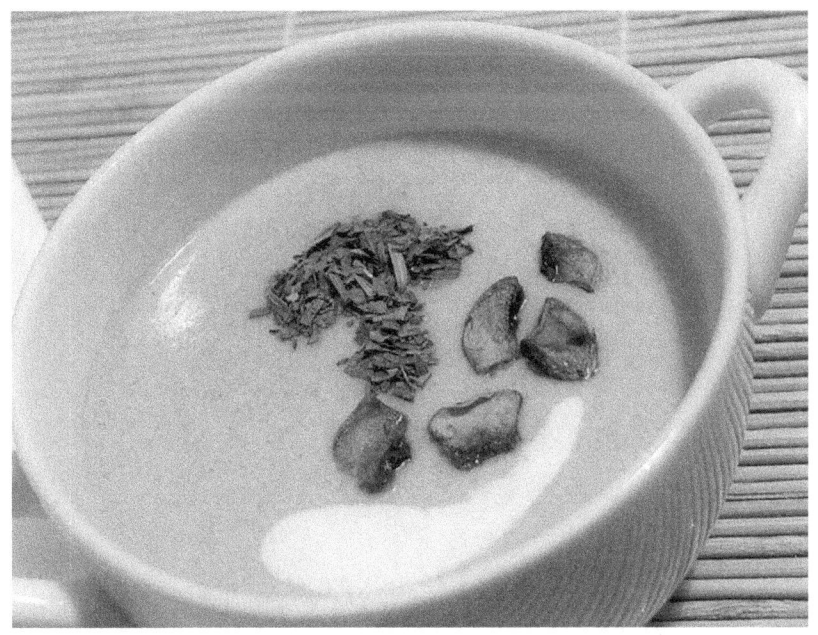

Serving Yields: 5
Nutritional Counts: Net Carbs: 6 g| Fat: 21 g

Ingredients:
- Olive oil – 1 tbsp.
- Diced onion - .5 of 1
- Sliced mushrooms – 20 oz.
- Minced cloves of garlic - 6
- Coconut cream – 1 cup
- Black pepper - .25 tsp.
- Sea salt - .75 tsp.
- Unsweetened almond milk – 1 cup
- Vegetable broth – 2 cups

Preparation Method:
1. Warm up a big cooking soup pot. Pour in the oil. Toss in the onions and mushroom. Sauté for 10-15 minutes. Fold in the garlic and cook for about one additional minute.
2. Fold in the remainder of the fixings and simmer until done (approx. 15 min.). Stir often.
3. Before serving, use an immersion blender until it's the desired consistency.

Red Onion Soup

Serving Yields: 2
Nutritional Counts: Net Carbs: 49.46 g| Fat: 51.91 g

Ingredients:
- Garlic cloves - 2
- Red onions - 2
- Lemon juice – 1.5 tbsp.
- Vegetable broth – 2.5 cups
- Olive oil – 5 tbsp.
- Walnuts – 4 tbsp.
- Low-carb bread – 2 slices
- Pepper and salt - to taste
- Pesto – 2 tsp.

Preparation Method
1. Slice the onions into ringlets and add to a saucepan and half of the oil. Toss in the minced garlic. Sauté for 5 minutes and add the juice and broth.
2. Sprinkle with the salt and pepper and simmer with the lid on the pot for 10 minutes.
3. Cube and fry the bread with the walnuts in the remainder of the oil until crispy.
4. Top off the hot soup with the walnuts, pesto, and croutons.

Spanish Soup

Serving Yields: 4
Nutritional Counts: Net Carbs: 6 g| Fat: 11 g

Ingredients:
- Tomatoes – 1.5 lb.
- Cucumber - 1
- White onion - .25 of 1
- Green bell pepper - .5 0 1
- Garlic-flavored olive oil – 3 tbsp.
- Black pepper and salt – as desired

Preparation Method:
1. Discard the pepper seeds and chop the cucumber, onion, peppers, and tomatoes. Combine the fixings in a food processor. Mix until smooth.
2. Cover and chill in the refrigerator for 1 hour. Serve with a few finely chopped peppers and tomatoes.

Spinach and Turnip Soup

Serving Yields: 2
Nutritional Counts: Net Carbs: 4.2 g| Fat: 13.3 g

Ingredients:
- Chopped turnips – 1.75 oz.
- Chopped spinach – 5.29 oz.
- Chopped ginger - .25 oz.
- Olive oil – 3 tsp.
- Desiccated coconut – approx. .33 oz.
- Coconut milk - .25 cup
- Water – 2 cups

Preparation Method:
1. Warm up the oil in a pan on the stovetop and sauté the ginger. Toss in the veggies and let it simmer over the high-temperature setting until the liquids are released.
2. Lower the heat and blend in the desiccated coconut.
3. Dilute the milk with the water and add to the pan. Simmer on the low heat setting.
4. When done, let it cool, and use an immersion blender to cream the soup.
5. Enjoy anytime.

Superfood Keto Soup

Serving Yields: 6
Nutritional Counts: Net Carbs: 6.8 g| Fat: 37.6 g

Ingredients:
- Medium head cauliflower – 1 – 14 oz.
- Medium white onion – 1
- Crumbled bay leaf – 1
- Garlic cloves – 2
- Frozen spinach – 7.8 oz of fresh spinach 7.1 oz. approx.
- Watercress – 5.3 oz.
- Vegetable broth – 1 liter
- Coconut milk – 8 fl. oz.
- Coconut oil - .25 cup
- Pink Himalayan rock salt – 1 tsp.
- Optional fresh herbs such as chives or parsley

Preparation Method:
1. Remove the skin from the onion and garlic. Dice them into fine bits.
2. Toss everything into a Dutch oven or soup pot - lightly greased with coconut oil. Simmer using the med-high heat setting until lightly browned.
3. Rinse the watercress and spinach. Sit to the side.
4. Dice the cauliflower into small florets and toss into the cooking pot with browned onion and crumbled bay leaf. Simmer for around five minutes.
5. Add the spinach and watercress and cook for another two to three minutes or until wilted. Pour in the vegetable stock and bring to a boil, cooking until the cauliflower is crisp-tender. Pour in coconut milk, adding a shake of

pepper and salt. Remove from the burner and pulse with a hand mixer.
6. Serve immediately or chill and keep refrigerated for up to five days.
7. You can also freeze for longer storage times.

Thai Pumpkin Soup

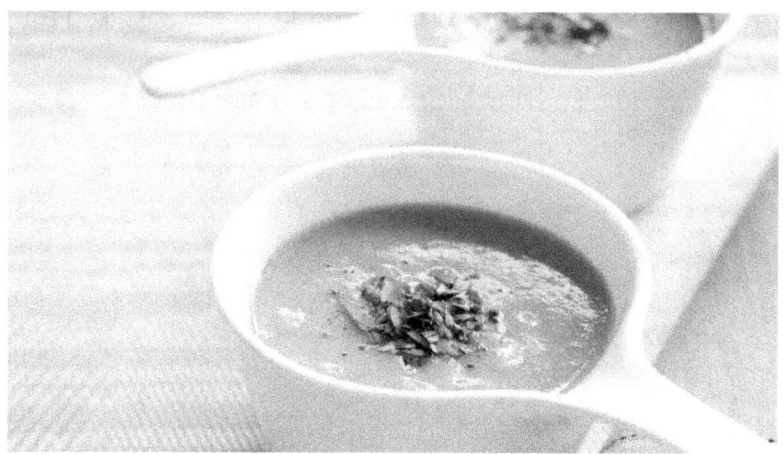

Serving Yields: 6
Nutritional Counts: Net Carbs: 11 g| Fat: 15 g

Ingredients:
- Sliced onion - 1
- Grated ginger – 1 tbsp.
- Pumpkin – peeled and chopped – 53 oz. approx.
- Coconut oil – 4 tsp.
- Mashed lemongrass - 1
- Thai red curry paste – 3 tbsp.
- Coconut milk – 1.75 cups
- Vegetable stock – 3.5 cups
- For Seasoning: Lime juice

Preparation Method:
1. Program the oven setting to 395°F.
2. Toss the cubes of pumpkin into 2 teaspoons of the oil and lime juice in a baking pan. Bake 30 minutes.

3. Warm up a skillet with the remainder of the oil and sauté the onion, lemongrass, and ginger for 8-10 minutes. Toss in the rest of the fixings and simmer for 5 more minutes.
4. Remove the lemongrass and cool. Mix well with an immersion blender before serving.

Turmeric Cabbage Soup

Serving Yields: 4
Nutritional Counts: Net Carbs: 5 g| Fat: 10 g

Ingredients:
- Coconut milk - .25 cup
- White cabbage – 1 head
- Turmeric powder – 2 tsp.
- Coconut oil – 2 tsp.
- Salt and pepper - .5 tsp. of each
- Cumin powder – 1 tsp.
- Vegetable stock – 3 cups
- Garlic cloves - 2

Preparation Method:
1. Peel and mince the garlic cloves.
2. Warm up a skillet and add the oil. Sauté the garlic and cabbage for 10 minutes.
3. Empty the stock into the mixture and simmer for 20 minutes (lid on).
4. Remove from the burner and stir in the rest of the fixings.
5. Prepare with an immersion blender until creamy smooth.
6. Tip: Turmeric is known for its health benefits, including fighting inflammation and is superb for those who suffer from arthritis.

Zucchini Basil Soup

Serving Yields: 4
Nutritional Counts: Net Carbs: 4 g| Fat: 7 g

Ingredients:
- Cloves of garlic – 2-3
- Zucchinis - 2
- Onion - 1
- Coconut oil – 2 tbsp.
- Basil leaves - .33 cup
- Pepper and salt - to taste
- Vegetable stock – 3 cups

Preparation Method:
1. Trim and chop the zucchini, cloves of garlic, and onion.
2. Warm the oil in a saucepan. When hot, toss in the onion and garlic. Sauté for 3 min.
3. Blend in the zucchini chunks and sauté another 5 min.
4. Empty the stock into the mixture and simmer 15 additional minutes.
5. At that time, mix in the basil.
6. Blend with an immersion blender until creamy.
7. Serve and enjoy.

Chapter 4: Vegan Creams - Sauces and Dips

Avocado Mayo

Serving Yields: 4
Nutritional Counts: Net Carbs: 4 g| Fat: 5 g

Ingredients:
- Avocado - .5 of 1 medium
- Pink salt – 1 pinch
- Ground cayenne pepper - .5 tsp.
- Lime juice - .5 of 1
- Olive oil - .25 cup

Preparation Method:
1. Dice the avocado and toss it into a blender or food processor. Pulse and add in the salt, cayenne, cilantro, and lime juice.
2. When smooth, stir in the oil – 1 tbsp. at a time - pulsing in between each addition.
3. You can store the mayo for up to one week in a sealed glass bottle.

Barbecue Sauce

Serving Yields: 2.5 cups – 2 tbsp. each

Ingredients:
- Agave nectar or pure maple syrup - 3 tbsp.
- Apple cider vinegar – 2 tbsp.
- Tomato sauce - 1 can – 15-16 oz.
- Molasses or extra syrup – 1 tbsp.
- Tamari - reduced-sodium soy sauce – 2-3 tbsp.
- Basil or dried oregano - 1 tsp.
- Chili powder - 1 tsp.
- Smoked or sweet paprika - 1 tsp.

Preparation Method:
1. Add all of the ingredients in a large container, whisking thoroughly.
2. Let it stand for one hour for all of the tasty flavors to blend fully.

Coconut Whipped Cream

Serving Yields: 8
Nutritional Counts: Net Carbs: 2.38 g| Fat: 10.4 g

Ingredients:
- Coconut cream – not the milk carton - 1 can
- Powdered sugar – vegan-friendly – 2-4 tsp.

Preparation Method:
1. Overnight: Refrigerate the cream.
2. Scoop the cream from the can – leaving the liquid behind. Use a mixer to beat 1 minute (high setting).
3. Add the sugar – to taste- and continue beating for another 4 minutes
4. Serve and enjoy chilled.

Eggplant Bruschetta

Serving Yields: 4
Nutritional Counts: Net Carbs: 2 g| Fat: 5 g

Ingredients:
- Eggplant - 1
- Olive oil – 2 tbsp.
- Salt - .5 tsp.
- Pepper – to taste

Ingredients for the topping:
- Chopped basil – 2 tbsp.
- Diced tomatoes – 2 cups
- Minced garlic cloves - 2
- Olive oil – 1 tbsp.
- Salt and Pepper – to your liking

Preparation Method:
1. Prepare the Veggies: Slice the eggplant in circles. Dice the tomatoes, chop the basil and mince the garlic cloves. Add to a salad bowl.
2. Sprinkle with the salt and set aside for ½ hour.
3. Grill the eggplant in a preheated grill (4-7 min. per side).
4. To serve, brush oil on the grilled eggplant slices and season to your liking.
5. Garnish with the topping and enjoy with your gang.

Guacamole

Serving Yields: 4
Nutritional Counts: Net Carbs: 5.4 g| Fat: 14.9 g

Ingredients:
- Cherry tomatoes – 7 oz.
- Avocados – 2
- White onion - 1
- Red chili pepper - 1
- Garlic cloves - 2
- Lime juice – 2 tbsp.
- Chopped cilantro – 2 tbsp.
- Salt and black pepper - to taste

Preparation Method:
1. Slice the avocados in half and scoop out the insides.
2. Mash and mix it with the rest of the fixings.
3. Serve any way you choose.

Hummus and Avocado

Serving Yields: 4
Nutritional Counts: Net Carbs: 2.4 g| Fat: 7.2 g

Ingredients:
- Lemon – juiced - .5 of 1
- Olive oil – 1 tbsp.
- Zucchini - 1
- Avocado - 1
- Creamy roasted tahini with salt - .25 cup
- Garlic cloves – minced - 3
- Sea salt – 1 tsp.
- Cumin – 1 tsp.

Preparation Method:
1. Peel and cube the zucchini and avocado. Mince the garlic cloves and add all of the fixings into a food processor. Mix until creamy smooth.
2. Let it chill in the fridge for 3-4 hours.
3. Serve and enjoy with the side of a veggie platter at your next dinner party!

Ketchup

Nutritional Counts: Net Carbs: 1 g| Fat: -0- g

Ingredients:
- Diced tomatoes – 1 can organic – 14.5 oz. (+) 1 can water
- Italian seasoning – 1 tsp.
- Star anise – 1 piece
- White vinegar - .5 tbsp.
- Freshly ground pepper
- Salt
- Optional: Erythritol – to your liking

Preparation Method:
1. Pour the tomatoes and a can of water into a small pan.
2. Stir in the herbs and anise. Simmer using the low heat setting for one hour, stirring frequently.
3. Transfer the pan from the heat and add the vinegar. Add any other seasonings as desired and remove the star anise.
4. Let it cool and puree into a smooth ketchup sauce using a blender/food processor.
5. Tip: Store in the fridge for no more than 4 days.

Lemon and Jalapeno Cream Sauce

Serving Yields: 8
Nutritional Counts: Net Carbs: 4.94 g| Fat: 7.08 g

Ingredients:
- Raw unsalted cashews - .75 cup
- Lemon juice – 5 tbsp.
- Lemon zest - .5 tsp.
- Fresh jalapeno - 1
- Olive oil - .5 tbsp.
- Cloves of garlic – skins-on - 2
- Unsweetened soy milk - .5 cup
- Salt - .5 tsp.

Preparation Method:
1. Heat up the oven setting to reach 400°F.
2. Soak the cashews for 2-4 hours in water. Line a baking sheet with some parchment paper.
3. Slice the jalapenos, remove the seeds, and place on the baking tin with the garlic cloves. Roast for 15 minutes.
4. Drain the cashews and add to a blender along with the oil, lemon juice, zest, salt, and soy milk. Toss in the peeled garlic cloves and jalapenos.
5. Puree and store in the refrigerator for up to seven days using a closed container.

Mayo – Vegan Style

Serving Yields: 1 cup – 1 tbsp. portions
Nutritional Counts: Fat: 13.8 g

Ingredients:
- Safflower oil – 1 cup
- Apple cider vinegar – 1 tsp.
- Unsweetened soy milk - .5 cup
- Juiced lemon - 1
- Sea salt - .75 tsp.

Preparation Method:
1. Use a high-speed blender to mix the lemon juice, soymilk, vinegar, and salt on the high-speed for one minute.
2. Slowly pour the oil while blending on low. (Remove the center lid cover.)
3. Blend on high with the lid back for about two minutes until thickened.
4. Add the mayonnaise to an airtight jar. It needs to chill for a minimum of one hour before using.

Nutella Spread

Serving Yields: 16
Nutritional Counts: Net Carbs: 3 g| Fat: 18.7 g

Ingredients:
- Roasted almonds - .5 cup
- Roasted hazelnuts – 1 cup
- Macadamia nuts – 1 cup
- Cacao powder -1 tbsp.
- Dark chocolate – 3.5 oz.
- Powdered erythritol – 2 tbsp.
- Virgin coconut oil - 1 tbsp.
- Vanilla powder - .5 tsp.

Preparation Method:
1. Mix the coconut oil and chocolate in a bowl. Melt using a water bath.
2. Use a food processor to turn the nuts into powder. Add the rest of the fixings and process until it reaches the desired texture.

Peanut Sauce

Serving Yields: 6
Nutritional Counts: Net Carbs: 6.4 g| Fat: 10.6 g

Ingredients:
- Ginger – 1- 5-inch piece
- Garlic cloves - 2
- Tamari - 2 tbsp.
- Water - .25 cup
- Lime juice – 1 tbsp.
- Red pepper flakes - .5 tsp.
- Stevia – 10 drops
- Chopped peanuts - .25 cup
- Chopped green onion – 2 tbsp.
- Natural peanut butter - .5 cup

Preparation Method:
1. Mix all of the fixings in a blender (omitting the onions and peanuts).
2. Mix until creamy and serve with the green onions and peanuts as a topping.

Portobello Mushroom Bruschetta

Serving Yields: 2
Nutritional Counts: Net Carbs: 2.48 g| Fat: 37.08 g

Ingredients:
- Minced garlic cloves - 6
- Portobello mushrooms - 2
- Olive oil – divided - .33 cup
- Chopped tomatoes - 3
- Chopped basil - .5 cup
- Pepper and Salt – to your liking

Preparation Method:
1. Combine 2 tbsp. of the oil with 2 garlic cloves in a cup.
2. Use a brush of the oil to season the mushrooms. Give the mushrooms a shake of the salt and pepper. Grill for 3 minutes (per side) using medium heat.
3. Prepare the basil and tomato mixture with the rest of the olive oil and garlic. Stuff the mushrooms and serve.

Slow-Cooked Summer Bruschetta

Serving Yields: 4
Nutritional Counts: Net Carbs: 7.5 g| Fat: 13 g

Ingredients:
- Quartered artichoke hearts - .5 cup
- Chopped basil leaves - 6
- Minced garlic – 2 tbsp.
- Capers - .25 cup
- Kalamata olives – halved - .25 cup
- Diced Roma tomatoes - 4
- Avocado oil - 3 tbsp.
- Balsamic vinegar - 3 tbsp.
- Sea salt - .75 tsp.
- Onion powder - .75 tsp.
- Ground black pepper - .5 tsp.

Preparation Method:
1. Combine all of the fixings in the cooker and mix well.
2. Prepare on the high setting for 3 hours. Be sure to stir 2-3 times during the cooking cycle.
3. Enjoy this tasty dish alongside your favorite grilled veggies.

Spinach Avocado Dip

Serving Yields: 12
Nutritional Counts: Net Carbs: 1.4 g| Fat: 8.8 g

Ingredients for the dip:
- Fresh spinach leaves - about 20 large leaves - .5 cup
- Ripened avocado – 2 large or about 2 cups of mashed
- Crushed garlic cloves – 1
- Freshly chopped coriander - .25 cup
- Dairy-free coconut or soy yogurt or another your choice - .75 cup
- Lime juice – 1 tbsp.
- Extra -virgin avocado oil or your favorite – 3 tbsp. (+) more to garnish
- Sea salt - .5 tsp.

Ingredients for the Mexican Salsa:

- Cherry tomatoes - a combo of colors yellow, red, or orange -10
- Chopped fresh coriander – 1 handful to taste
- Ex.-virgin avocado oil – 2 tbsp.
- Lime juice – 1 tbsp.
- Clove of garlic - 1
- Brown Rice Chips – 1 pkg.

Preparation Method:
1. Trim the fresh spinach leaves. Blanche the leaves by placing them into a large mixing bowl and cover with

boiling water. Place a lid on the dish and set aside for two minutes.
2. Rinse the spinach using cold water. Squeeze the cooked/blanched spinach leaves to remove all the extra water. Pat them dry on two sheets of absorbent paper towels to remove all the extra water.
3. In a food processor, with 'S' blade attachment, add the spinach, mashed ripened avocado, crushed garlic, coriander, coconut yogurt, lime juice, avocado oil, salt, and pepper.
4. Process until smooth - about two minutes using the high-speed setting. Transfer into a bowl. Drizzle oil on top if you like.
5. Refrigerate at least 30 minutes before serving or before adding the Mexican salsa.
6. It stores well in the fridge for up to one week in an airtight container. The surface of the dip may change slightly in color - avocado oxidation - simply give a good stir and enjoy.

Preparation Method for the Salsa:
1. In a mixing bowl, add the chopped tomatoes.
2. Combine with avocado oil, crushed garlic, and lime juice.
3. Sprinkle the salsa on top of the dip with extra chopped coriander.
4. Serve with a pack of brown rice chips.
5. **Tips: Oil Options:** If you don't have avocado oil, any vegetable oil works well. The healthiest alternative will be extra virgin olive oil.

Tahini and Cilantro Sauce

Serving Yields: 4
Nutritional Counts: Net Carbs: 4.97 g| Fat: 9.64 g

Ingredients:
- Minced garlic cloves - 2
- Tahini - .33 cup
- Water - .25 cup
- Fresh cilantro - .5 cup
- Apple cider vinegar – 1 tbsp.
- Salt - .25 tsp.
- Lemon juice – 1 tsp.

Preparation Method:
1. Squeeze the lemons for fresh juice.
2. Combine all of the components in a blender. Puree and flavor to taste.
3. Note: You can refrigerate the sauce for up to two weeks.

Tofu or Seitan Marinades

Enjoy the Variety:

Serving Yields: 2 – each marinade is enough for 1 block of tofu or 2 seitan tenders

Ingredients:
BBQ Marinade:
- BBQ sauce - check to make sure it's vegan – 6 tbsp.
- Liquid smoke - .5 tsp.

Coconut Curry Marinade:
- Full-fat coconut milk - .5 cup
- Curry powder – 2 tsp.
- Soy sauce – 2 tbsp.

Jerk Marinade:
- Jerk marinade (hot, mild, or a combo) – 3 tbsp.
- Water – 2 tbsp.

Italian Marinade:
- White wine vinegar or Lemon juice – 2 tbsp.
- Olive oil - 2 tbsp.
- Dried rosemary – 1 tsp.
- Dried basil – 1 tsp.
- Garlic powder - .25 tsp.
- Salt - .25 tsp
- Black pepper - .125 tsp.

Lemon Mustard Marinade:

- Lemon juice – 2 tbsp.
- Dijon mustard – 2 tbsp.
- Maple syrup or agave – 1 tbsp.
- Black pepper - .125 tsp.

Sriracha Marinade:
- Sriracha – 2 tbsp.
- Soy sauce or substitute – 1 tbsp.
- Agave or maple syrup - 1 tbsp.

Sweet Chili Marinade:
- Sweet chili sauce - .25 cup
- Soy sauce – 1 tbsp.

Balsamic Marinade:
- Olive oil – 2 tbsp.
- Garlic powder - .5 tsp.
- Balsamic vinegar – 2 tbsp.

Thai Peanut Marinade:
- Peanut butter – 3 tbsp.
- Lime juice – 1.5 tbsp.
- Soy sauce – 1.5 tbsp.
- Agave – 2 tsp.
- Garlic powder - .5 tsp.
- Powdered ginger - .5 tsp.

Mexican Marinade:
- Light oil – 2 tbsp.

- Lime juice – 2 tbsp.
- Agave – 1 tbsp.
- Chili powder – 2 tsp.
- Smoked paprika – 1 tsp.
- Garlic powder - .5 tsp.

Sweet and Smoky Marinade:
- Olive oil – 2 tbsp.
- Maple syrup or agave – 2 tbsp.
- Soy sauce – 2 tbsp.
- Liquid smoke – 1 tsp.
- Garlic powder - .5 tsp.
- Chili powder - .5 tsp.

Teriyaki Marinade:
- Brown sugar – 2 tbsp.
- Soy sauce or substitute – 2 tbsp.
- Orange juice or water – 2 tbsp.
- Garlic powder - .5 tsp.
- Powdered ginger - .5 ts
- p.

Instructions for the marinades:
1. For any marinade you choose, simply add all of the ingredients to a resealable bag or airtight container.
2. Mix and add your seitan tenders or sliced/cubed tofu.
3. Let them marinate for a minimum of 15 minutes or up to 4 days.

Vegan Sour Cream

Serving Yields: Just over 1 cup
Nutritional Counts: Net Carbs: 1 g| Fat: 1 g

Ingredients:
- Extra-firm silken or crumbled firm tofu – 1 cup
- Rice milk – as needed – 2-3 tbsp.
- Lemon juice – 2 tsp. or to taste
- Salt - .25 tsp or as desired

Preparation Method:
1. Mix all of the components in the blender or food processor. Puree until smooth.
2. Store in an airtight container.

Veggie Salsa

Serving Yields: 4
Nutritional Counts: Net Carbs: 4.9 g| Fat: 13.8 g

Ingredients:
- Cherry tomatoes – 2 cups
- Cucumber - 1
- Red onion - .5 of 1
- Lime juice - 2 tbsp.
- Chopped parsley - 2 tbsp.
- Garlic cloves - 2
- Extra-virgin olive oil - .25 cup
- Pepper and Salt – as desired

Preparation Method:
1. Peel and dice the cucumber. Dice the rest of the veggies and mince the garlic.
2. Toss all of the components into a serving dish. Enjoy as a side at your next party.

Chapter 5: Appetizers – Sides and Snacks

Sides

Basil Zoodles and Olives

Serving Yields: 6
Nutritional Counts: Net Carbs: 8.4 g| Fat: 41.7 g

Ingredients:
- Fresh basil - .5 cup
- Spiralized zucchini – 4
- Avocado pesto - .5 cup
- Kalamata olives – 1 cup
- Drained sun-dried tomatoes - .25 cup
- Sliced avocados – 2
- Coconut oil – extra-virgin – 2 tbsp.
- Salt - .25 tsp.

Preparation Method:
1. Remove the pits and drain the olives as you drain the tomatoes. Slice the avocados into strips.
2. Spritz a pan with the coconut oil and prepare the noodles for two to five minutes – in batches if needed.
3. Mix the pesto and noodles in a mixing container. Toss in the rest of the fixings and serve.

Beetroot and Pesto Noodles

Serving Yields: 1
Nutritional Counts: Net Carbs: 13 g| Fat: 21 g

Ingredients:
- Beetroots - 2

Pesto Ingredients:
- Lime juice – 1 tsp.
- Avocado - 1
- Red chili pepper - 1
- Clove of garlic - 1

Preparation Method:
1. Prepare the Fixings: Peel, spiralize, and lightly steam the beetroots. Peel and finely mince the garlic clove. Remove the seeds from the pepper and chop finely.
2. Combine all of the pesto components.
3. Toss the prepared noodles with the pesto and enjoy.

Brussels Sprouts and Cashew Dip

Serving Yields: 10
Nutritional Counts: Net Carbs: 11.6g| Fat: 17 g

Ingredients:
- Trimmed Brussels sprouts – 1 lb.
- EVOO – 2 tbsp.
- Pepper - .25 tsp.
- Salt - .5 tsp.

Ingredients for the dip:
- Minced clove of garlic - 1
- Unsweetened Silk Cashew Milk – 1 cup
- Lemon juice – 3 tbsp.
- Unsweetened cashew butter – 1.5 cup
- Black pepper – 2 tsp.
- Coarse sea salt - .5 tsp.

Preparation Method:
1. Set the oven temperature at 400°F.
2. Toss the sprouts in a baking pan with the oil, pepper, and salt.
3. Bake for 12-15 minutes. Set aside.
4. Combine the dip fixings in a blender, mixing until smooth.
5. Enjoy as a side dish at any time.

Cabbage Slaw

Serving Yields: 2
Nutritional Counts: Net Carbs: 7 g| Fat: 33 g

Ingredients:
- Shredded green cabbage – 4 cups
- Tamari – 2 tbsp.
- Minced garlic cloves - 2
- Sesame oil – 1 tbsp.
- Vinegar – 1 tsp.
- Chili paste – 1 tsp.
- Chopped Macadamia nuts - .5 cup

Preparation Method:
1. Toss the fixings (omit the nuts) into a skillet using the low setting.
2. Prepare covered for about 5 minutes. Stir in the nuts and continue cooking for another five minutes.
3. Serve and enjoy to complement any meal.

Carrot and Zucchini Noodles in Thai Sauce

Serving Yields: 2
Nutritional Counts: Net Carbs: 9 g| Fat: 26 g

Ingredients:
- Carrot - 1
- Zucchini - 1
- Coconut milk - .5 cup
- Thai curry paste – 1 tbsp.
- Coconut oil – 2 tbsp.
- Also Needed: 1 Wok

Preparation Method:
1. Peel and spiralize the carrot and zucchini.
2. Warm up a wok and add the oil. Prepare the zucchini and carrots for 3-5 minutes.
3. Combine the paste and milk. Stir in with the noodles.
4. Continue to cook for another 30 seconds or so.

Cauliflower and Artichoke Couscous

Serving Yields: 4
Nutritional Counts: Net Carbs: 8 g| Fat: 9 g

Ingredients:
- Black olives - 16
- Trimmed – riced - cauliflower head - 1
- Artichokes – 1 jar – 14 oz.
- Lemon – zest and juice - 1
- Olive oil – 2 tbsp.
- Black pepper and salt – .5 tsp.
- Parsley - .25 cup
- Clove of garlic - 1

Preparation Method:
1. Finely chop the garlic and parsley after you trim the cauliflower head.
2. Prepare a baking tray and toss it with the oil while adding the cauliflower.
3. Bake at 400°F for 12 minutes. Toss about halfway through the cooking cycle.
4. Fold in the rest of the fixings and enjoy.

Cauliflower Bites with Ranch Dip

Serving Yields: 8
Nutritional Counts: Net Carbs: 2.4 g| Fat: 27.9 g

Ingredients:
- Cauliflower florets – 4 cups
- Garlic powder - .25 tsp.
- Salt - .25 tsp.
- Smoked paprika - .25 tsp.
- Extra-virgin olive oil – 2 tbsp.
- Sugar-free hot sauce - .5 cup

Ingredients for the dip:
- Unsweetened coconut milk - .5 cup
- Freshly squeezed lemon juice – 1 tbsp.
- Organic dairy-free mayo – 1 cup
- Garlic powder – 1 tsp.
- Pepper - .25 tsp.
- Onion powder – 1 tsp.
- Fresh parsley - .25 cup

Preparation Method:
1. Whisk the ingredients for the dip and place in the fridge.
2. Mix the hot sauce with the garlic powder, salt, and paprika. Toss in the cauliflower. Shake and then spread it in the prepared pan.
3. Bake for 30 minutes.
4. Serve with bites with the dip anytime you have a get-together with friends and family.

Cherry Tomatoes and Zucchini Pasta

Serving Yields: 4
Nutritional Counts: Net Carbs: 13.1 g| Fat: 24 g

Ingredients:
- Thinly sliced red onion - 1
- Spiralized zucchini – 2 lb.
- Halved cherry tomatoes – 1 pint
- Minced cloves of garlic - 4
- Chopped basil - .5 cup
- EVOO - .25 cup
- Pepper and salt – as desired
- Crushed red pepper - .5 tsp.
- For the Topping: Shredded parmesan

Preparation Method:
1. Warm up the oil in a pot. Sauté the garlic and onion. Toss in the zucchini, pepper, and salt. Cook 2 minutes, stirring once.
2. Toss in the tomatoes and cook for 3-4 minutes. Then, add the basil and red pepper.
3. Garnish with the cheese and serve.

Chili and Coconut Cauliflower Rice

Serving Yields: 3
Nutritional Counts: Net Carbs: 4.6 g| Fat: 7.3 g

Ingredients:
- Full-fat coconut milk - .66 cup
- Riced cauliflower – 1 pkg.
- Onion powder - .5 tsp.
- Salt – as desired
- Chili paste – 1 tsp.
- Fresh basil – garnish

Preparation Method:
1. Combine all of the components in a saucepan.
2. Cook with the lid on for about 5-10 minutes. Stir every minute or so to prevent sticking.
3. Take the lid off and continue cooking until it has absorbed the liquid.

Coconut Cauliflower Rice

Serving Yields: 6
Nutritional Counts: Net Carbs: 3.1 g| Fat: 6.9 g

Ingredients:
- Full-fat coconut cream – 1 cup
- Chopped cauliflower - .5 of 1 head
- Cilantro – 1 tsp.
- Unsweetened shredded coconut - .25 cup
- Salt – to your liking

Preparation Method:
1. Use a food processor to rice the cauliflower.
2. Use the medium heat setting to warm a pan.
3. Add all of the fixings and simmer until softened.
4. Stir occasionally and serve when tender. It shouldn't take more than five minutes to prep and about ten minutes of cooking time for a delicious side dish.

Creamy Curry Low-Carb Noodle Bowl

Serving Yields: 4
Nutritional Counts: Net Carbs: 7.3 g| Fat: 15.4 g

Ingredients:

- Kanten Noodles – 1 pkg.
- Carrots – julienned - 2
- Cauliflower - roughly chopped - .5 of 1 head
- Red bell pepper - diced - 1
- Freshly chopped cilantro – 1 handful
- Mixed greens – 2 handfuls
- Dairy-free creamy curry sauce – 1 batch
- Water – Approx. 2 cups

Preparation Method:

1. Prepare the Kanten Noodles by placing the two sheets of noodles in a large bowl. Lightly heat the water, a couple of degrees below boiling. Think of it as hot water that you can drink.
2. Pour water over the noodles and set aside while you prepare the rest of the ingredients. After about 5 minutes of soaking, strain and set aside in a large bowl to cool.
3. Add carrots, cauliflower, bell pepper, and cilantro to the bowl with the noodles. Set mixed greens on 2 separate servings plates as the "base" to your meal.
4. Then, prepare the Creamy Curry Sauce.
5. Serve immediately or place in the fridge to cool for a couple of hours. Store in an air-tight container in the fridge for up to 2 days.

For the creamy sauce:

Serving Yields: 4
Nutritional Counts: Net Carbs: 2.8 g| Fat: 15.2 g

Ingredients:
- Avocado oil or MCT oil – 2 tbsp.
- Tahini or avocado oil mayo - .25 cup
- Water - .25 cup
- Apple cider vinegar – 2 tbsp.
- Ground coriander – 1.5 tsp.
- Curry powder - 2 tsp.
- Sea salt – 1 tsp.
- Freshly-cracked black pepper - .5 tsp.
- Turmeric – 1 tsp.
- Cumin – 1 tsp.
- Ground ginger - .25 tsp.

Preparation Method:
1. Combine all of the fixings into the jug of a high-powered blender.
2. Pulse until smooth.
3. Add the veggie and noodle mixture and toss to coat.

Edamame Kelp Noodles

Serving Yields: 2
Nutritional Counts: Net Carbs: 4.9 g| Fat: 8.6 g

Ingredients:
- Kelp noodles – 1 pkg.
- Frozen spinach – 1 cup
- Shelled edamame - .5 cup
- Julienned carrots - .25 cup
- Sliced mushrooms - .25 cup

Ingredients for the sauce:
- Sesame oil - 1 tbsp.
- Tamari – 2 tbsp.
- Garlic powder - .5 tsp.
- Ground ginger - .5 tsp.
- Sriracha - .25 tsp.

Preparation Method:
1. Prepare the noodles in a pan of water to soak. Drain well.
2. Combine the sauce components in a pan using the medium heat setting.
3. Toss in the vegetables.
4. Once the mixture is hot, toss in the soaked noodles.
5. Simmer and stir occasionally with a lid on until steamy hot.

Garlicky Mushrooms

Serving Yields: 3
Nutritional Counts: Net Carbs: 5 g| Fat: 8 g

Ingredients for Step # 1:
- Minced garlic cloves - 4
- Cremini mushrooms - 24 oz.
- Bay leaves - 2
- Dried oregano - .5 tsp.
- Dried basil - .5 tsp.
- Dried thyme - .25 tsp.
- Vegetable broth – 1 cup
- Black pepper and salt – to your liking
- Unsalted butter – 2 tbsp.
- Half and Half - .25 cup
- Parsley – 2 tbsp.

Preparation Method:
1. Mix all of the fixings (step 1) in a slow cooker and prepare using the low setting for 3-4 hours.
2. About 20 minutes before it's done, combine the butter and Half and Half for the sauce.
3. Garnish with freshly chopped parsley and enjoy.

Grilled Eggplant and Zucchini

Serving Yields: 2
Nutritional Counts: Net Carbs: 6 g| Fat: 14 g

Ingredients:
- Eggplants - 2
- Zucchinis - 2
- Garlic cloves - 2
- Parsley - 2 tbsp.
- Mint - 2 tbsp.
- Olive oil – 4 tsp.
- Erythritol – 1 tbsp.
- Red wine vinegar – 4 tsp.
- Pepper and salt – to taste

Preparation Method:
1. Slice the zucchini and eggplants lengthwise. Chop the veggies.
2. Brush the eggplant and zucchini with the oil. Sprinkle with salt and pepper.
3. Place on a hot griddle pan and brown on both sides. Place on the serving dish.
4. Warm up the rest of the oil and sauté the garlic. Add the erythritol and vinegar. Pour over the veggies and garnish with the mint and parsley.

Indian Curried Cauliflower

Serving Yields: 4
Nutritional Counts: Net Carbs: 5 g| Fat: 7 g

Ingredients:
- Peanut oil – 2 tbsp.
- Cauliflower - .5 of 1 head - chopped
- Cumin seeds – 1 tsp.
- Chopped shallots - .5 cup
- Pepper and salt -to taste
- Sweet curry – 1.5 tsp.
- Chopped cilantro - .25 cup
- Lime – juiced - 1

Preparation Method:
1. Warm up a 'wide' pan and sauté the seeds for about 30 seconds.
2. Toss in the shallots, cauliflower, pepper, salt, and curry powder. Cook for 7-8 minutes – stirring occasionally.
3. Toss in the cilantro. Serve with a drizzle of lime juice.

Kelp Noodles with Peanut Butter Sauce

Serving Yields: 4
Nutritional Counts: Net Carbs: 2 g| Fat: 16 g

Ingredients:
- Kelp Noodles
- White onion – 1
- Garlic cloves – 3
- Peanut butter - .5 cup
- Soy sauce – keto-friendly - .25 cup
- Lime juiced – 1
- Red pepper flakes – 2 tsp.

Preparation Method:
1. Soak the kelp noodles in water and drain.
2. Combine all of the sauce fixings in a blender. Mix well until creamy.
3. When ready to serve, just add the sauce on top of the noodles. Enjoy.

Lime and Chili Carrot Noodles

Serving Yields: 1
Nutritional Counts: Net Carbs: 4 g| Fat: 27 g

Ingredients:
- Jalapeno chilis - 2
- Carrots - 2
- Lime juice - 1 tbsp.
- Coconut oil - 2 tbsp.
- Coriander - .25 cup
- Black pepper - .5 tsp.
- Salt - .5 tsp.

Preparation Method:
1. Prepare the vegetables. Deseed and finely chop the jalapenos. Peel and spiralize the carrots and finely chop the coriander.
2. Combine the oil, lime juice, and jalapeno. Toss and add the carrots.
3. Blend in the rest of the fixings and serve.

Mediterranean Spaghetti Squash

Serving Yields: 4
Nutritional Counts: Net Carbs: 14.77 g| Fat: 22.91 g

Ingredients:
- Spaghetti squash - 1
- Pine nuts – 2 tbsp.
- Pesto - .25 cup
- Kalamata olives - .33 cup
- Freshly chopped basil - .25 cup
- Cherry tomatoes - 10
- Cremini mushrooms – 10 oz.
- Salt and pepper – as desired
- Olive oil – as needed

Preparation Method:
1. Set the oven temperature to 400°F. Cover a baking sheet with parchment paper.
2. Slice the squash -lengthwise- and remove the seeds. Drizzle with the oil, pepper, and salt. Place in the pan (cut side down) and bake for 30-40 minutes. Let it rest for about 10 minutes.
3. Meanwhile, add the mushrooms to a parchment paper-lined pan. Give them a splatter of oil, salt, and pepper. Bake until browning begins (10-15 min.).
4. Using the medium heat setting to combine the pesto and squash in a large skillet. Cook for 3-4 minutes until the squash is slightly crispy.
5. Lower the heat (medium) and add the rest of the fixings. Cook for another 5-10 minutes; stir frequently and season to your liking.

Mushroom, Broccoli, and Squash Noodles

Serving Yields: 1
Nutritional Counts: Net Carbs: 5.4 g| Fat: 17.51 g

Ingredients:
- Broccoli florets - .5 cup
- Spiralized summer squash - 1
- Chopped almonds - 5
- Halved cherry tomatoes - 5
- Olive oil – 1 tbsp.
- Sliced cremini mushrooms - 5
- Parsley pesto – 2 tbsp.

Preparation Method:
1. Warm up a skillet with the oil. When hot, toss in the mushrooms. Add the florets of broccoli and stir for about 2 minutes (half cooked).
2. Add the squash 'noodles' and stir for another 2 minutes.
3. Transfer to the countertop and add the rest of the fixings.

Nutty Pesto Zucchini

Serving Yields: 2
Nutritional Counts: Net Carbs: 11.46 g| Fat: 26.08 g

Ingredients:
- Basil leaves - 5
- Zucchinis – ribbon slices - 3
- Salt - .5 tsp.
- Olive oil – 1 tbsp.
- Parmesan cheese - .25 cup

Ingredients for the Pesto:
- Walnuts - .25 cup
- Peeled garlic cloves - 2
- Avocado - .5 of 1
- Water – if necessary - .5 of a cup
- Fresh basil leaves – 1 cup
- Lemon - .5 of 1

Preparation Method:
1. After slicing the zucchini, sprinkle it with the salt, and set aside for now.
2. Use a blender and add the pesto components – blending until smooth. Add water if needed.
3. Warm up the oil in a pan and simmer the zucchini for 4 minutes.
4. Transfer to a platter with the pesto. Sprinkle with the cheese and basil before serving.

Pesto Kelp Noodles

Serving Yields: 3
Nutritional Counts: Net Carbs: 1.3 g| Fat: 32.7 g

Ingredients:
- Kelp noodles – 1 pkg.

Pesto Ingredients:
- Baby spinach leaves – 1 cup
- Haas avocado – 1 pitted
- Cloves of garlic - 2
- EVOO - .5 cup
- Basil - .25 cup
- Salt – 1 tsp.

Preparation Method:
1. Rinse and soak the noodles for about 30 minutes.
2. Mix the pesto fixings in a blender until creamy smooth.
3. Drain and toss the noodles into about ¼ cup of the sauce. Save the rest for another time!

Roasted Beetroot Noodles

Serving Yields: 3
Nutritional Counts: Net Carbs: 10 g| Fat: 25 g

Ingredients:
- Baby kale – 2 cups
- Spiralized beets - 2

Ingredients for the Pesto:
- Pine nuts - .25 cup
- Olive oil - .25 cup
- Basil leaves – 3 cups
- Ground black pepper - .5 tsp.
- Ground sea salt - .5 tsp.
- Minced garlic clove - 1

Preparation Method:
1. Prepare a baking tin with a layer of non-stick cooking spray.
2. After spiralizing the noodles, give them a dusting of pepper and salt.
3. Heat up the oven to 425ºF. Prepare for 5 minutes or to your liking.
4. Combine the pesto fixings in a food processor until smooth.
5. Toss it all together and enjoy.

Roasted Broccoli

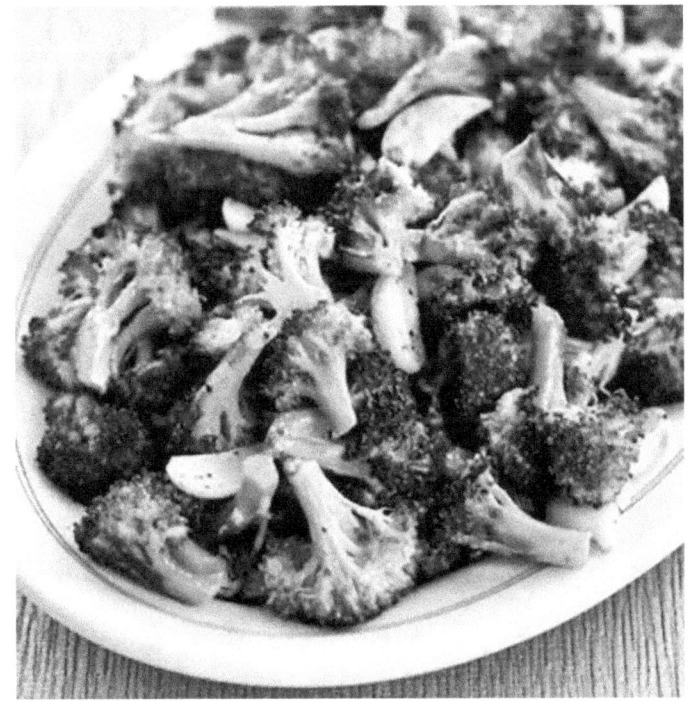

Serving Yields: 4
Nutritional Counts: Net Carbs: 7 g| Fat: 14.3 g

Ingredients:
- Extra-virgin olive oil - .25 cup
- Broccoli – 2 - into florets
- Salt - .5 tsp.
- Minced garlic cloves - 2

Preparation Method:
1. Incorporate all of the fixings and add them to a baking dish.

2. Set the oven temperature to reach 450°F. When hot, add the prepared veggies to the oven and bake for 15 minutes.
3. Serve for a luncheon treat or dinner side dish.

Roasted Green Cabbage

Serving Yields: 2
Nutritional Counts: Net Carbs: 9 g| Fat: 21 g

Ingredients:
- Green cabbage head - 1
- Garlic cloves - 4
- Olive oil – 4 tbsp.
- Pepper and salt – as desired

Preparation Method:
1. Peel and mince the garlic cloves. Remove the outer leaves of the cabbage and slice the remainder into 6-inch slices. Add the slices to a baking sheet.
2. Brush the fixings with oil and about half of the garlic. Give it a sprinkle of salt and pepper.
3. Set the oven to 400°F. Prepare for 20 minutes. Flip the cabbage and sprinkle with the rest of the garlic. Continue baking for 20 more minutes.
4. Serve piping hot!

Roasted Kale and Squash

Serving Yields: 8
Nutritional Counts: Net Carbs: 10 g| Fat: 35 g

Ingredients:
- Torn kale – 2 tbsp.
- Spaghetti squash – 1
- Chili powder - .5 tsp.
- Pepper and salt- to taste
- Balsamic vinegar – 1 tsp.
- Diced onion - .5 of 1
- Olive oil – as needed

Preparation Method:
1. Remove the seeds and cut the squash into halves. Place it cut side up on a baking sheet. Cover it with some of the oil.
2. Prepare the oven setting to 350°F. Bake until done.
3. Meanwhile, add 1 tbsp. of oil to a skillet and sauté the onion for about 3 minutes. Add to the kale with a shake of salt and pepper. Bake for another 5 minutes.
4. Remove the squash strands and add the vinegar, a tbsp. of oil, and the chili powder. Serve together and enjoy.

Spaghetti Squash

Serving Yields: 4
Nutritional Counts: Net Carbs: 4 g | Fat: 7 g

Ingredients:
- Olive oil – 2 tbsp.
- Spaghetti squash 1 whole
- Sage - .5 tsp.
- Cracked pepper - .5 tsp.
- Salt – 1 tsp.
- Dried parsley – 1 tsp.
- Garlic powder – 1 tsp.
- Dried rosemary – 1 tsp.
- Dried thyme – 1 tsp.
- Also needed: Baking pan

Preparation Method:
1. Set the oven temperature to 350°F.
2. Cut the squash in half and discard the seeds. Add some water to the baking tin and add the squash – cut side downwards.
3. Roast for 45 minutes to 1 hour.
4. Remove and cool. Scoop out all of the flesh and add to a mixing bowl with the rest of the fixings.
5. Cook for another 15 minutes before serving.

Sriracha Grilled Asparagus

Serving Yields: 4
Nutritional Counts: Net Carbs: 3.75 g| Fat: 17 g

Ingredients:
- Trimmed asparagus – 1 lb.
- Kosher salt - to taste
- Olive oil – 1 tsp.

Ingredients for the sauce:
- Avocado oil - .25 cup
- Sriracha sauce - 1 tbsp.
- Lime juice - 1 tbsp.
- Vegan-friendly tamari – 2 tsp
- Rice wine vinegar – 2 tbsp.
- Granulated sugar-free sweetener – your choice – 1 tsp.

Preparation Method:
1. Toss the salt, oil, and asparagus together. Place on the grill and cook until tender.
2. Prepare the sauce. Whisk the fixings (not the pecans). Then, blend in the pecans.
3. Pour the sauce over the grilled asparagus and serve it to your waiting guests.

Teriyaki Grilled Eggplant

Serving Yields: 5
Nutritional Counts: Net Carbs: 6.98 g| Fat:12.07 g

Ingredients:
- Cloves of garlic - 2
- Medium eggplants - 2
- Sesame oil - .25 cup
- Liquid aminos - .5 cup
- Ground ginger – 1 tbsp.
- Granulated swerve – 2 tbsp.
- Toasted sesame seeds – 1 tbsp.

Preparation Method:
1. Peel and crush the garlic cloves. Use the medium heat setting and combine the garlic, sesame oil, liquid aminos, swerve, and ginger into a saucepan.
2. Once it is gently simmering, continue frequently stirring until it begins to thicken slightly. Take it off of the burner and set aside for now.
3. Warm up the grill. Remove the stems from the eggplants. Cut into slices about 1/8-inch thick. Brush each eggplant slice with the teriyaki sauce and place it on the grill.
4. Sear each side, brushing with more sauce as it caramelizes. Top it off with a portion of the sauce and some toasted sesame seeds.

Tofu Pizza Sticks

Serving Yields: 4
Nutritional Counts: Net Carbs: 3.8 g| Fat: 5.7 g

Ingredients:
- Extra-firm tofu – 1 block
- Tomato sauce - .25 cup (+) 1 tbsp.
- Nutritional yeast – 2 tbsp. (+) 2 tsp.
- Dried basil – 1-2 pinches

Preparation Method:
1. Drain the Tofu: Wrap the block of tofu in a paper towel. Weigh down something heavy on top to press. Let the tofu drain for about 15-20 minutes.
2. Warm up the oven to reach 425°F. Prepare a cookie sheet with a layer of parchment paper.
3. Slice the tofu into 16 thin pieces and arrange in the pan. Spread the sauce on each of the sticks. Sprinkle with the nutritional yeast and a dusting of the basil to taste.
4. Bake for 27-30 minutes

Turnip Fries

Serving Yields: 6
Nutritional Counts: Net Carbs: 4.4 g| Fat: 9.5 g

Ingredients:
- Organic turnips – 2 lb.
- Taco seasoning – 2 tbsp.
- Unrefined sea salt - .5 tsp.
- Light olive oil - .25 cup

Preparation Method:
1. Set the oven temperature at 350°F.
2. Peel and chop the turnips (chip-thin). Combine all of the fixings in a Ziploc-type baggie and shake well.
3. Prepare a baking tin with parchment paper and add the fries.
4. Bake until golden – tossing about halfway through (25 min.).

Turnip and Courgette Hash Browns

Serving Yields: 1
Nutritional Counts: Net Carbs: 8 g| Fat: 12 g

Ingredients:
- Courgetti – grated with moisture removed - .5 cup
- Grated turnip – 1 cup
- Grated onion – 1
- Garlic powder – 1 tsp.
- Pepper and salt – to taste
- Olive oil – 2 tbsp.
- Fresh thyme – 1 tbsp.

Preparation Method:
1. Combine all of the fixings except for the olive oil.
2. Warm up the oil in a skillet. Toss in small portions of the mixture.
3. Simmer until golden brown and flip. Finish cooking the second side.
4. Continue until done and serve.

Zucchini Noodles and Avocado Sauce

Serving Yields: 2
Nutritional Counts: Net Carbs: 9 g| Fat: 26.8 g

Ingredients:
- Zucchini - 1
- Basil - 1.25 cups
- Water - .33 cup
- Avocado - 1
- Pine nuts – 4 tbsp.
- Sliced cherry tomatoes - 12
- Lemon juice – 2 tbsp.

Preparation Method:
1. Use a spiralizer or a veggie peeler to prepare the zucchini noodles.
2. Combine the remainder of the fixings (except the tomatoes) in a blender until creamy smooth.
3. Mix together the avocado sauce, noodles, and cherry tomatoes in a mixing container.
4. You can enjoy these delicious noodles stored in the refrigerator for one or two days.

Snack Time Treats

Carrot Cake Bites

Serving Yields: 15
Nutritional Counts: Net Carbs: 1 g| Fat: 1 g

Ingredients:
- Coconut flour - .5 cup
- Water - .5 cup (+) 1 tbsp.
- Unsweetened applesauce – 2 tbsp.
- Vanilla extract - .5 tsp.
- Cinnamon – 1 tsp.
- Granulated Lakanto Monk Fruit Sweetener - 4 tbsp.
- Carrot - 1 medium
- Reduced fat shredded coconut – 4 tbsp.

Preparation Method:
1. Combine the coconut flour, applesauce, water, and v anilla extract in a large mixing bowl. Stir well.
2. Finely shred or chop the carrot. Add in cinnamon, Lakanto, and shredded carrots to a bowl, and stir to combine. Refrigerate dough for 15 minutes.
3. Place the shredded coconut in a small bowl.
4. After 15 minutes, remove dough from fridge and roll into 15 cake balls. Roll each ball in shredded coconut until evenly coated.
5. Store in refrigerator for up to a week.
6. Tip: You can use another granulated sweetener of choice, equivalent to 4 tablespoons of sugar.

Chocolate Granola

Serving Yields: 32
Nutritional Counts: Net Carbs: 4.2 g| Fat: 17.5 g

Ingredients:
- Unsweetened cocoa - .125 cup
- Melted coconut oil – 1.8 oz.
- Granulated sweetener – your favorite – 2 tbsp.
- Cinnamon – 1 tsp.
- Pumpkin seeds – 3.5 oz.
- Shredded coconut – 3.5 oz.
- Sunflower seeds – 3.5 oz.
- Chopped almonds – 3.5 oz.
- Flaxseeds – 3.5 oz.
- Chopped walnuts – 3.5 oz.

Preparation Method:
1. Warm the oven to reach 350°F.
2. Combine the sweetener, cinnamon, coconut oil, and cocoa.
3. Toss the seeds, coconut, and all of the nuts in a baking dish and add the mixture from (step 2). Stir well.
4. Bake for 20 minutes until browned and crispy. Toss every 4 minutes.

Chocolate Protein Bars

Serving Yields: 8
Nutritional Counts: Net Carbs: 1.4 g | Fat: 13.9 g

Ingredients:
- Raw hemp hearts - .75 cup
- Raw sunflower seeds - .5 cup
- Cocoa powder - .25 cup
- Chia seeds - .25 cup
- Psyllium husk powder – 2 tbsp.
- Salt - .5 tsp.
- Liquid stevia - .25 tsp.
- Water – 1 cup

Preparation Method:
1. Preheat the oven temperature to 250°F.
2. Grind the seeds to a flour-like texture. Combine with the dry fixings.
3. Add the water – as you stir - to form a thick dough. Spread the batter on a baking sheet to a 1-inch thickness.
4. Bake for 1 1/2 hours.
5. Divide the bars into eight servings and bake for another 15 minutes.
6. Serve or enjoy anytime.

Cinnamon Granola

Serving Yields: 4
Nutritional Counts: Net Carbs: 3.74 g| Fat: 19.08 g

Ingredients:
- Unsweetened coconut flakes - 5 tbsp.
- Ground flax meal - 5 tbsp.
- Chia seeds – 1 tbsp.
- Sugar-free maple syrup – 4 tbsp.
- Nuts – walnuts, pecans, etc. – 1.5 oz.
- Cinnamon – 1.5 tsp.

Preparation Method:
1. Prepare a baking sheet with a layer of baking parchment paper. Heat the oven to 350°F.
2. Combine everything (omit the cinnamon) in a mixing bowl.
3. Mix well and spread out over the baking tin with a sprinkle of the cinnamon– single layer.
4. Bake, stirring once, for 20-22 minutes.
5. Remove and let the granola harden. Store using an airtight bowl.

Coconut and Peanut Butter Balls

Serving Yields: 15
Nutritional Counts: Net Carbs: 0.92 g| Fat: 3.19 g

Ingredients:
- Unsweetened coconut powder – 3 tsp.
- Creamy peanut butter – vegan-friendly – 3 tbsp.
- Almond flour – 2 tsp.
- Powdered erythritol – 2.5 tsp.
- Coconut flakes - .5 cup

Preparation Method:
1. Combine the cocoa, flour, peanut butter, and erythritol. Mix well and freeze for 1 hour. Use a small spoon to scoop out the mixture.
2. Drop it into the flakes of coconut. Roll it around with your hand and refrigerate overnight for the best firming results.

Fudge Balls

Serving Yields: 12
Nutritional Counts: Net Carbs: 7.4 g| Fat: 28.8 g

Ingredients:
- Unsweetened cocoa powder - .5 cup
- Almond, peanut, or cashew nut butter – 1 cup
- Coconut oil – 1 cup
- Coconut flour - .33 cup
- Pink Himalayan salt – 1 pinch
- Monk fruit sweetener - .5 to 1 tsp. or .25 tsp. powdered stevia

Preparation Method:
1. Combine the chosen nut butter and add it and the coconut oil in a saucepan (med. heat). Stir in the rest of the fixings.
2. Freeze in a glass dish for 20 minutes until it's firmed up somewhat.
3. Remove and form into 1-inch balls. You must work quickly, or the oil will melt.
4. Return to the freezer for 10-15 minutes. Store in a closed container in the freezer.

Loaded Nut-Packed Coconut Granola

Serving Yields: 20
Nutritional Counts: Net Carbs: 5.9 g| Fat: 18.5 g

Ingredients:
- Unsweetened coconut flakes - .5 cup
- Raw pecans – 1.25 cups
- Raw walnuts – 1 cup
- Raw almonds – 2 cups
- Chia seeds - 3 tbsp.
- Ground cinnamon – 1.5 tsp.
- Sea salt - .25 tsp.
- Flaxseed meal – 1 tbsp.
- Coconut sugar – 2 tbsp.
- Maple syrup - .25 cup (+) 1 tbsp.
- Coconut oil - 3 tbsp.
- Roasted – unsalted – Sunflower seeds - .25 cup
- Dried blueberries - .25 cup

Preparation Method:
1. Prepare the oven temperature to 325°F.
2. Combine the coconut sugar, nuts, coconut, flaxseed meal, salt, and cinnamon in a mixing container.
3. Warm up the maple syrup and coconut oil using the medium heat setting (stovetop). Pour into the mixture (Step 1).
4. Add the fixings to the baking sheet and spread as evenly as possible.
5. Bake in the preheated oven for 20 minutes.
6. Transfer to the countertop. Stir in the blueberries and sunflower seeds.

7. Bake for another 5-8 minutes at 340°F.
8. Transfer from the oven and set on a cooling rack to cool.

Mushroom Chips

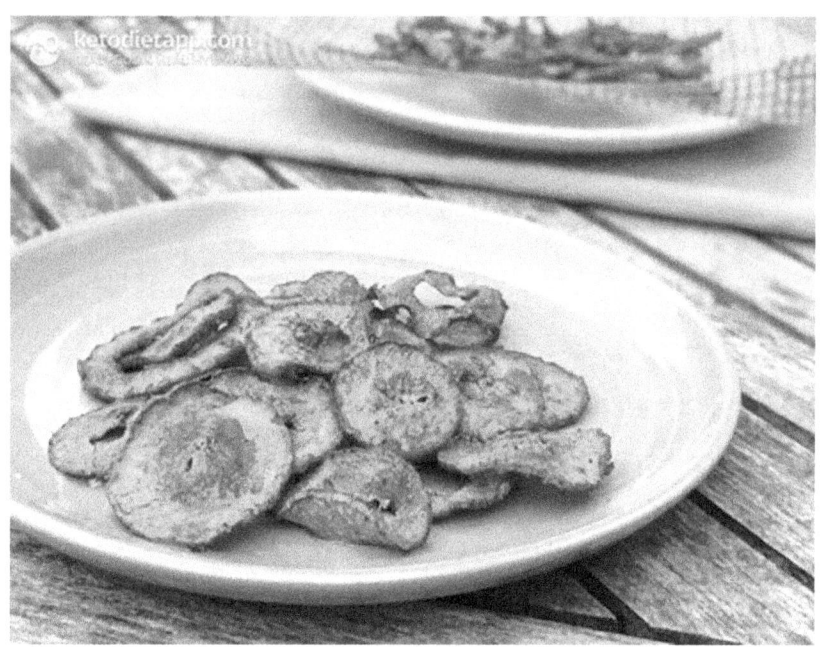

Serving Yields: 4
Nutritional Counts: Net Carbs: 3.8 g| Fat: 15.5g

Ingredients:
- Coconut oil – 4 tbsp.
- Portobello mushrooms – 10.6 oz.
- Salt - .5 tsp.
- Dash- Ground black pepper

Preparation Method:
1. Brush a little oil on the baking sheet.
2. Slice the mushrooms thin and add to the prepared tin.
3. Sprinkle with the pepper and salt and bake at 300°F for 45-60 minutes.
4. Flip 2-3 times during the process for even browning.

Pecan and Maple Fat Bars

Serving Yields: 12
Nutritional Counts: Net Carbs: 2 g| Fat: 30.5 g

Ingredients:
- Halved pecans – 2 cups
- Almond flour – 1 cup
- Golden flaxseed meal - .5 cup
- Shredded coconut – unsweetened - .5 cup
- Coconut oil - .5 cup
- Liquid stevia - .25 tsp.
- Maple syrup – keto friendly - .25 cup

Preparation Method:
1. Program the oven setting to 350°F. Add the pecans to a pan and toast for 6-7 minutes. Cool and crush in a plastic bag.
2. Combine all of the dry components – including the pecans. Stir in the wet ingredients to form a crumbly dough. Spread it onto a baking dish and press. Prepare in the hot oven for 20-15 minutes.
3. Take the bars out of the oven to cool for 15-20 minutes. Next, place in the fridge for about 1 hour until cold.
4. Serve and enjoy any time.

Peanut Butter Fat Bombs

Serving Yields: 24
Nutritional Counts: Net Carbs: 2.4 g| Fat: 8.7 g

Ingredients:
- Extra-virgin coconut oil - .5 cup
- Peanut Butter - smooth style, with salt -- sugar-free - .5 cup
- Trader Joes Coco Powder unsweetened 3 serving or 1 tbsp.
- Vanilla extract - .5 tsp
- Pyure Organic Stevia all-purpose sweetener - 9 tsp.
- NOW MCT Oil – 2 tbsp.
- Jif Powdered Peanut Butter - 2 tbsp.

Preparation Method:
1. Melt your coconut oil and your peanut butter. Then, mix using a hand mixer. Next, add the coco powder and your vanilla. Mix - scraping the sides as needed.
2. For the Pyure, you will want to adjust to your sweetness liking. It will need to be ground in a coffee grinder to give it a powdered sugar texture.
   Then pour it into the bowl. Mix well and add the powdered PB and the CT and mix again.
3. Pour into ice cube tray and store in the freezer compartment of the fridge until set for about one hour. Then, you can store them in the fridge in a container. Use parchment paper to separate layers if you stack them.

Peanut Tofu Wrap

Serving Yields: 4
Nutritional Counts: Net Carbs: 5 g| Fat: 12 g

Ingredients:
- Crumbled extra-firm tofu – 1 pkg. 16 oz.
- Savoy cabbage leaves - 4 Large
- Canola oil – 1 tbsp.
- Prepared peanut sauce – 5 tbsp.
- Salt - .25 tsp.
- Rice vinegar – 1 tbsp.
- Julienned Asian pear – 1 cup
- Lime zest – 1.5 tsp.
- Julienned English cucumber – 1 cup
- Cilantro – finely chopped - .25 cup

Preparation Method:
1. Cut the cabbage crosswise and into halves. Crumble the tofu.
2. Warm up a skillet and add the oil. Sauté the tofu for 4-6 minutes (seasoned with salt) until lightly browned.
3. Whisk the peanut sauce, vinegar, and zested lime. Take the pan from the burner and mix the sauce. Toss well.
4. Add the tofu fixings to each of the cabbage pieces.
5. Garnish with the cilantro, pear, and cucumber. Serve.

Roasted Radish Chips

Serving Yields: 4
Nutritional Counts: Net Carbs: 1.2 g| Fat: 7.1 g

Ingredients:
- Radishes – 16 oz.
- Pepper and salt - .5 tsp. of ea.
- Coconut oil – 2 tbsp.

Preparation Method:
1. Chop the radishes into thin rounds. Toss all of the fixings together.
2. Bake – single-layered – at 400°F for 12-15 minutes.
3. Enjoy for a quick and tasty treat anytime.

Sweet Potato Toast

Serving Yields: 4
Nutritional Counts: Net Carbs: 9.02 g| Fat: 23.85 g

Ingredients:
- Ripe avocado - 1
- Large sweet potato - 1
- Pepper and salt – as desired
- Roughly-chopped pistachios - .5 cup
- Olive oil – 3 tbsp.
- Crushed red pepper flakes - optional

Preparation Method:
1. Warm up the oven to 400°F. Prepare a baking sheet with aluminum foil.
2. Slice the potato into 1/4-inch rounds. Arrange on the baking sheet and toss it with the oil, salt, and pepper.
3. Bake for 20 minutes and garnish with the avocado and pistachios. Add a few pepper flakes.

Zucchini Chips

Serving Yields: 8
Nutritional Counts: Net Carbs: 2.3 g| Fat: 3.6 g

Ingredients:
- Zucchini – 4 cups
- Coarse sea salt – 2 tsp.
- EVOO – 2 tbsp.
- White balsamic vinegar – 2 tbsp.

Preparation Method:
1. Cover a baking pan with parchment paper.
2. Thinly slice the zucchini. Whisk the oil and vinegar together and toss with the zucchini.
3. Arrange the zucchini on the baking tin in an even layer. Give it a sprinkle of salt.
4. Bake at 200°F for 2-3 hours. Flip about halfway through the cooking process. Enjoy any time.

Chapter 6: Desserts – Smoothies and Beverages

Pudding Specialties

Avocado and Chocolate Pudding

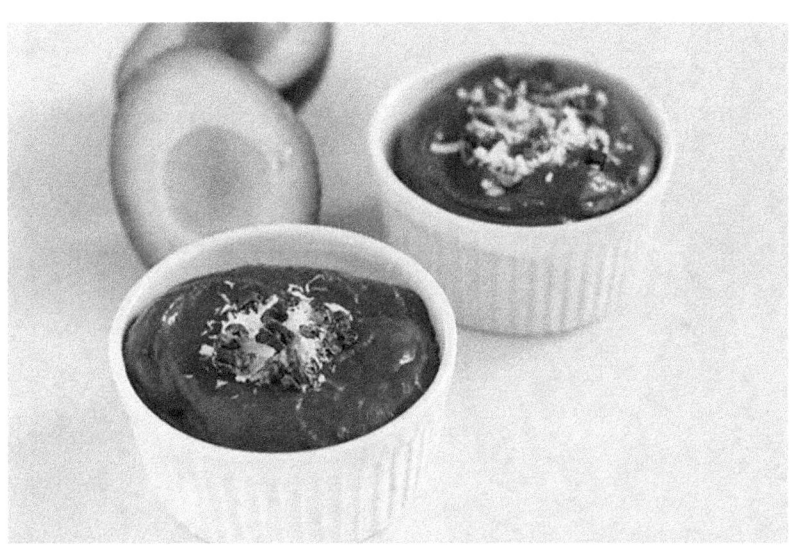

Serving Yields: 1
Nutritional Counts: Net Carbs: 6 g| Fat: 24 g

Ingredients:
- Avocado – pit removed - 1
- Cocoa powder - .25 cup
- Pink salt – 1 tsp.
- Vanilla extract - .5 tsp.
- Stevia – 10 drops

Preparation Method:
1. Combine the fixings in a mixing bowl. Beat well with a fork. Continue whipping until it is as you like it!
2. Chill and serve.

Chia Chocolate Pudding

Serving Yields: 8
Nutritional Counts: Net Carbs: 14.9 g| Fat: 16.5 g

Ingredients for Day 1:
- Vanilla extract – 1 tsp.
- Coconut milk – 2 cups
- Unsweetened cocoa powder - .25 cup
- Maple syrup - .25 cup
- Salt – 1 pinch
- Chia seeds - .66 cup

Ingredients for Day 2:
- Unsweetened shredded coconut - 1 tbsp.
- Coconut milk- 1 tbsp.
- Optional: Whipped cream - 1 tbsp.
- Coconut sugar – 1 tsp.

Preparation Method:
1. Day 1 Prep: Whisk all of Day 1's ingredients, adding the chia seeds last. Add the mixture to a large jar with a lid to combine for about five minutes.
2. Gently rotate the jar for 30 seconds and rest for four minutes. Continue for 20 more minutes. Place the mixture in the fridge overnight or at least for eight hours.
3. Day 2 Prep: Add the pudding into a mixing container and blend the ingredients (omit the milk).
4. Drizzle with 1 tbsp. of coconut milk over the top of the pudding.
5. Garnish as desired.

Chia Raspberry Pudding

Serving Yields: 4
Nutritional Counts: Net Carbs: 4.3 g| Fat: 18.2 g

Ingredients:
- Coconut milk – 1 cup
- Water - .5 cup
- Fresh raspberries – 1 cup
- Whole chia seeds - .5 cup
- Vanilla powder – 1 tsp.

Preparation Method:
1. Mix the raspberries, milk, and water in a blender until smooth.
2. Fold in the chia seeds and vanilla.
3. Chill the pudding overnight for best results.

Chia Strawberry Pudding

Serving Yields: 1
Nutritional Counts: Net Carbs: 11 g| Fat: 57 g

Ingredients:
- Stevia – 1 dash
- Chopped strawberries - .25 cup
- Chia seeds – 2 tbsp.
- Vanilla essence - .5 tsp.
- Coconut milk – 1 cup

Preparation Method:
1. Combine the ingredients in a canning jar with a lid. Close the top and shake well.
2. Store in the refrigerator for at least eight hours. Enjoy this treat anytime!

Coconut Chia and Turmeric Pudding

Serving Yields: 1
Nutritional Counts: Net Carbs: 14 g| Fat: 78 g

Ingredients:
- Chia seeds – 2 tbsp.
- Coconut milk – 6 oz.
- Ground cardamom - .25 tsp.
- Unsweetened desiccated coconut - .5 cup
- Peeled and grated turmeric – 1 piece – 1-inch
- Also Needed: 1 mason jar

Preparation Method:
1. Mix all of the fixings in a mason jar and close the top.
2. Shake the jar to mix well and let the goodies steep overnight in the fridge.
3. Wake up to a ready-to-go meal for one of those fast-moving mornings.

Pumpkin and Peanut Butter Pudding

Serving Yields: 2
Nutritional Counts: Net Carbs: 13 g| Fat: 61 g

Ingredients:
- Pumpkin puree - .5 cup
- Peanut Butter – keto-friendly - .5 cup
- Chia seeds – 2 tbsp.
- Coconut milk – 1 cup

Preparation Method:
1. Measure out and all of the fixings into a blender.
2. Give the container a quick blitz and pour into a mason jar.
3. Place in the fridge to chill; overnight, preferably.

Other Delicious Desserts

Avocado Chocolate Mousse

Serving Yields: 3 generous portions
Nutritional Counts: Net Carbs: 19 g| Fat: 27 g

Ingredients:
- Chopped semisweet chocolate – 4 oz. *or* at least 60% dark chocolate chips – or about .5 cup (+) 2 tbsp.
- Large ripe avocados - 2 - 8 oz. ea.
- Kosher salt - .125 tsp.
- Unsweetened cocoa powder – 3 tbsp.
- Unsweetened Almond Breeze Blend - .25 cup
- Pure vanilla extract – 1 tsp.
- Optional: Light agave nectar 1–3 tsp. - pure maple syrup
- For Serving: Sliced strawberries or fresh raspberries - whipped coconut cream, and a few chocolate shavings

Preparation Method:
1. Use a microwave-safe and toss in the chips of chocolate. Melt for 15 seconds at a time, mixing well. Stir well and set aside to cool.
2. Slice the avocado and remove the pit. Add to a food processor along with the cocoa powder, salt, melted chocolate, milk blend, and vanilla extract. Continue blending, scraping the sides until creamy smooth.
3. Adjust the sweetness with a few teaspoons of the agave as desired.

4. Spoon into glasses and enjoy immediately as a pudding or for a thicker, mousse-like consistency. For best results, chill overnight or a minimum of two hours.
5. Serve topped with raspberries, cream, and chocolate shavings.

Banana Bread

Serving Yields: 12
Nutritional Counts: Net Carbs: 4 g| Fat: 8 g

Ingredients:
- Blanched almond flour – 2 cups
- Granulated sweetener of choice – 2 tbsp.
- Cinnamon - 1 tsp.
- Baking powder – 1 tsp.
- Salt - .25 tsp.
- Large overripe bananas, mashed – 2
- Flax eggs –2 - replacement for 2 regular hen eggs
- Coconut oil - .5 cup
- Vanilla extract – 1 tsp.

Preparation Method:
1. Warm up the oven to reach 350°F. Grease a loaf pan or 10 x 10-inch square pan and set to the side.
2. Combine the dry fixings in a mixing container, mixing well. In a separate bowl, melt your coconut oil. Add your mashed bananas and flax eggs/eggs and whisk together.
3. Combine all of the fixings (dry and wet) and toss until entirely incorporated. Pour into the greased pan. Bake for 40-50 minutes.
4. Note: A square pan tends to be around the 40-minute mark, whereas a loaf pan is at the 45-50-minute mark or until a toothpick comes out clean from the center.
5. Cool the cake in the pan for ten minutes. Then, move it to cool onto a wire rack. Slice and serve.

Cashew and Blueberry Cheesecake

Serving Yields: 8
Nutritional Counts: Net Carbs: 6 g| Fat: 16 g

Ingredients for the crust:
- Cinnamon – 1 tsp.
- Desiccated coconut – 2 tbsp.
- Ground flaxseeds – 2 tbsp.

Ingredients for the filling:
- Soaked cashews – 1 cup
- Vegan-type cream cheese – 4 oz.
- Lemon juice – 1 tbsp.
- Coconut oil – 2 tbsp.
- Frozen blueberries - .5 cup
- Vanilla extract – 1 tsp.
- Liquid stevia – to your liking

Preparation Method:
1. Mix all of the crust components and flatten using two containers.
2. Combine all of the filling fixings in a blender until smooth.
3. Empty the filling into the containers and chill until firm.
4. Serve anytime you want a yummy treat.

Chilled Avocado and Strawberry Bowl

Serving Yields: 1
Nutritional Counts: Net Carbs: 5 g| Fat: 10 g

Ingredients:
- Lime – 1 tsp.
- Peeled – pitted – avocado – 1 cup
- Pinch of salt – 1 pinch
- To Your Liking: Stevia

Preparation Method:
1. Combine all of the goodies in a blender.
2. Incorporate until smooth and place in the fridge to chill.

Cinnamon and Pumpkin Fudge

Serving Yields: 25 servings
Nutritional Counts: Net Carbs: 2.19 g| Fat: 10.63 g

Ingredients:
- Ground nutmeg - .25 tsp
- Ground cinnamon – 1 tsp.
- Pumpkin puree – 1 cup
- Warmed/melted coconut butter – 1.75 cups
- Coconut oil – 1 tbsp.

Preparation Method:
1. Combine the fixings (coconut butter, spices, and pumpkin). Whisk in the coconut oil.
2. Spread the mixture over a foil-lined baking dish and cover with wax paper. Press out the fudge until even. Discard the paper and place in the fridge for 2 hours.
3. Chop into squares and keep handy for the next sugar craving!

Coconut Bombs

Serving Yields: 30
Nutritional Counts: Net Carbs: 1 g| Fat: 13 g

Ingredients:
- Coconut oil - .75 cup
- Coconut milk – 1 can
- Unsweetened coconut flakes – 1 cup
- Liquid stevia – 20 drops

Preparation Method:
1. Add the oil to a microwavable bowl. Let it cook for about 20 seconds or until melted. Stir in the stevia and milk.
2. Add the coconut flakes and pour into candy molds.
3. Place in the freezer for one hour. Yummy!

Coconut Cupcakes

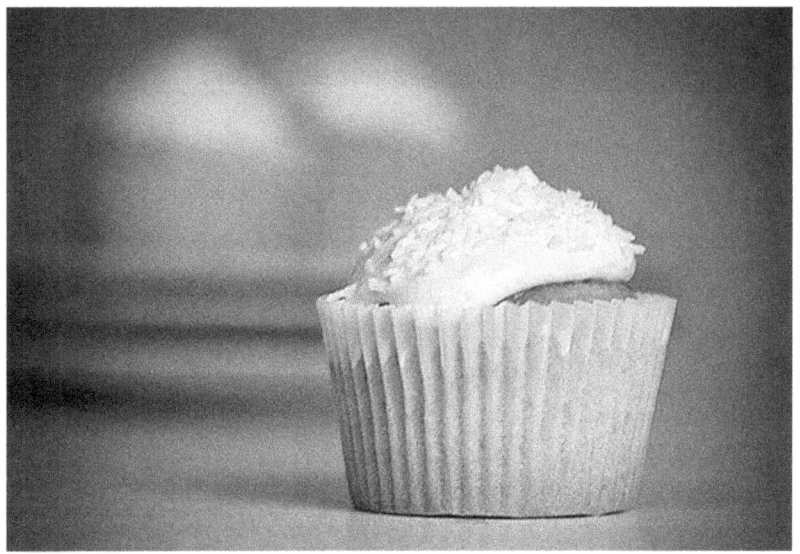

Serving Yields: 7
Nutritional Counts: Net Carbs: 4.25 g| Fat: 30.7 g

Ingredients:
- Psyllium husk – 2 tbsp.
- Vanilla flavored protein powder – 4.25 oz.
- Unsweetened coconut flakes – 3 oz.
- Coconut oil – 4 tbsp.
- Unsweetened coconut milk – 6.7 oz.
- 85% cocoa – dark chocolate - .75 oz.

Preparation Method:
1. Combine the coconut flakes, psyllium, and protein powder. Mix and blend in the coconut milk and oil. Add the mixture into cupcake forms.

2. Melt the chocolate in a saucepan and drizzle the cupcakes.
3. Freeze for about 30 minutes and sprinkle with the pecan halves.
4. Let them firm up in the refrigerator for 2 hours.
5. Cut into pieces and enjoy.
6. Add a delicious low-carb frosting if desired, but count the extra carbs.

Coconut Maple Fudge

Serving Yields: 18
Nutritional Counts: Net Carbs: 0.5 g| Fat: 9.1 g

Ingredients:
- Coconut oil - .5 cup
- Coconut butter - .5 cup
- Maple extract – 1 tsp.
- Shredded – unsweetened- toasted coconut - .5 cup
- Liquid stevia coconut sweet drops - .5 tsp.

Preparation Method:
1. Add a layer of parchment paper to a baking tin.
2. Melt the coconut butter and oil in a pan (low heat). Combine everything (Omit the coconut for now.).
3. Sprinkle the coconut on the prepared baking sheet. Pour the batter over the mixture.
4. Place in the refrigerator to firm up. Then, cut into 18 pieces and enjoy!

Coconut and Peanut Butter Balls

Serving Yields: 15
Nutritional Counts: Net Carbs: 0.92 g| Fat: 3.19 g

Ingredients:
- Unsweetened cocoa powder – 3 tsp.
- Creamy peanut butter – vegan-friendly – 3 tbsp.
- Almond flour – 2 tsp.
- Powdered erythritol – 2.5 tsp.
- Unsweetened coconut flakes - .5 cup

Preparation Method:
1. Combine the cocoa, peanut butter, erythritol, and flour.
2. Place in the freezer for 1 hour.
3. Using a small spoon, prepare the servings and drop them into coconut flakes.
4. Roll them around and reshape if needed.
5. Refrigerate until firm.

Coconut and Strawberry Bars

Serving Yields: 2
Nutritional Counts: Net Carbs: 4 g| Fat: 28 g

Ingredients:
- Melted coconut butter – 16 oz.
- Coconut oil – 1 tbsp.
- Chopped strawberries – 1 cup
- Coconut – dry- .25 cup
- Stevia – 1 tsp.

Preparation Method:
1. Combine the butter, oil, and stevia to make the bowl have a 'greasy' appearance. Add the berries and garnish with the coconut.
2. Place in the fridge for four hours. When chilled, cut into bars.
3. Enjoy anytime you want a tasty treat.

Dairy-Free Chocolate Silk Pie

Serving Yields: 8
Nutritional Counts: Net Carbs: 6.6 g| Fat: 41.31 g

Ingredients:
- Chilled coconut milk, liquid discarded – 2 cans - 13.5-oz. each
- Almond butter - .5 cup
- Vanilla extract – 1 tsp.
- Granulated erythritol - .25 cup
- Low-carb dark chocolate – 4 oz.
- Almond flour – 1 cup
- Coconut flour – 2 tbsp.
- Granulated sweetener – 2 tbsp.
- Xanthan gum – 1 tsp.
- Sea salt - .5 tsp.
- Ghee – 2 tbsp.
- Water – 1-2 tbsp.
- Slivered almonds -for the garnish – 2 tbsp.

Preparation Method:
1. In a saucepan, heat the coconut cream, sweetener, vanilla, and almond butter until they're completely melted together.
2. Take the saucepan off of the burner. Stir until the chocolate is melted and creamy smooth. Refrigerate the mixture while you prepare the crust.
3. Whisk or sift the flours, sweetener, salt, and xanthan gum. Using a fork, cut in the ghee until the mixture is crumbly and beginning to resemble dough.

4. Add half of the water and knead into dough. If it's looking dry, add more water so the mixture is sticky to the touch.
5. Press into a pie tin and bake at 350°F for 15 minutes or until the edges brown. Once the crust is baked, pour the chocolate filling into the pie tin and place in the freezer for at least 4 hours.
6. Slice the pie and serve cold. Refrigerate any leftovers!

Lime Avocado Popsicles

Serving Yields: 6
Nutritional Counts: Net Carbs: 3.2 g| Fat: 21.9 g

Ingredients:
- Erythritol - .25 cup
- Coconut milk – 1.5 cups
- Avocados - 2
- Lime juice – 2 tbsp.

Preparation Method:
1. For a tasty treat on a hot day, simply dice the avocados into chunks and add them with the rest of the fixings to a blender. Mix until smooth.
2. Pour the mixture into six popsicle molds and gently tap the container on the countertop to remove any air bubbles.
3. Freeze for 7-8 hours with a stick inserted in the center of the mold.
4. Run water over the mold to remove the delicious popsicle.

Mexican Chocolate Avocado Ice Cream

Serving Yields: 6 (3 cups)
Nutritional Counts: Net Carbs: 4.16 g| Fat: 25.74 g

Ingredients:
- Full-fat coconut milk - 15- oz. – 1 can
- Swerve Sweetener - .33 cup
- Espresso powder - optional – 1 tsp.
- Sugar-free - chopped dark chocolate – ex. Lily's – 3 oz.
- Vanilla extract – 1 tsp.
- Medium California Avocados – 2
- Ground cinnamon – 1.5 tsp.
- Chipotle powder - .25 to .75 tsp. - depending on how spicy you like it

Preparation Method:
1. Whisk together the sweetener and espresso powder with the milk in a pan until the sweetener has dissolved. The expresso will post the flavor of the chocolate.
2. Chop the chocolate. Take the saucepan off of the burner and add the chocolate. Let it cool for about four until chocolate is melted, then whisk in the vanilla - mixing until smooth.
3. Combine the cinnamon, chipotle chocolate mixture, and avocados in a blender or food processor. Puree until smooth.
4. Store in the fridge for at least two hours. Transfer into an ice cream maker and churn until the consistency resembles soft serve ice cream (this takes less time than custard-based ice creams).

5. Serve as soft serve or transfer to an airtight container and freeze another few hours for a firmer consistency.

Minty Berries in A Dish

Serving Yields: 6
Nutritional Counts: Net Carbs: 8.5 g| Fat: 12 g

Ingredients:
- Full-fat coconut milk – 1 can
- Freshly chopped mixed berries – 4 cups
- Vanilla pod – seeds only – 1 pod
- Birch xylitol - 1 tsp.
- Fresh mint leaves - 1

Preparation Method:
1. Mix the mint and berries in a mixing container.
2. Empty the liquid from the coconut and throw it away. Place the 'hard' coconut in a bowl with the vanilla seeds.
3. Using a hand mixer, mix the vanilla mixture and stevia.
4. Serve the berries and cream for breakfast or a luscious dessert.

Pecan and Blueberry Crumble

Serving Yields: 6
Nutritional Counts: Net Carbs: 15.24 g| Fat: 31.33 g

Ingredients:
- Chia seeds – 3 tbsp.
- Lemon juice – 1 tbsp.
- Blueberries – 14 oz.
- Stevia powder – 1.5 tsp.
- Blanched almond flour – 2 cups
- Cinnamon – 2 tbsp.
- Chopped pecans - .25 cups
- Coconut oil – 5 tbsp.

Preparation Method:
1. Warm up the oven to 400°F.
2. Prepare a cast iron skillet. Combine the berries, stevia, chia seeds, and lemon juice. Pour into the pan.
3. Mix the rest of the fixings in a bowl and spread over the pan of berries.
4. Add the skillet to the hot oven and bake for 30 minutes.
5. Remove and portion out to six servings.

Pumpkin Truffles

Serving Yields: 18
Nutritional Counts: Net Carbs: 1.4 g| Fat: 6.1 g

Ingredients:
- Pumpkin spice – 2 tsp.
- Pumpkin puree – 1.5 cups
- Softened coconut butter - .75 cup
- Vanilla extract – 1 tsp.
- Vanilla liquid stevia – 1 tsp.

Preparation Method:
1. Prepare a baking sheet with a piece of parchment paper.
2. Add all of the fixings in a blender. Once it's creamy, use a scoop and add the truffles to the baking tin.
3. Place in the refrigerator until firm. Enjoy anytime!

Raspberry Coconut Bark

Serving Yields: 12
Nutritional Counts: Net Carbs: 2.45 g| Fat: 23.56 g

Ingredients:
- Frozen berries - .5 cup
- Coconut oil - .5 cup
- Coconut butter - .5 cup
- Unsweetened shredded coconut - .5 cup
- Powdered Swerve sweetener - .25 cup

Preparation Method:
1. Line a baking tin with parchment paper.
2. Turn the frozen berries into powder with a food processor. Set aside.
3. Mix the rest of the fixings in a saucepan (low heat). Stir until melted.
4. Pour ½ of the mixture into the baking pan.
5. Mix the rest of the pan mixture with the powdered berries (step 2). Stir well and spoon the raspberry delight over the coconut mix and swirl with a butter knife.
6. Place in the freezer until it can be easily broken into pieces (bark).

Raspberry Truffles

Serving Yields: 24
Nutritional Counts: Net Carbs: 5.4 g| Fat: 10.8 g

Ingredients:
- Fresh raspberries – 1 cup
- Unsweetened cashew butter – 1 cup
- Melted coconut oil – 2 tbsp.
- Raspberry extract - .5 tsp.
- Berry liquid stevia - .5 tsp.
- 85% dark chocolate – 1 - 8 oz. portion
- Salt – 1 pinch

Preparation Method:
1. Line a baking sheet with a sheet of baking parchment paper
2. Mix all of the fixings - but omit the chocolate for now - in a food processor and pulse until smooth.
3. Scoop out 24 truffles and press a raspberry in the center of each. Place on the prepared cookie sheet and freeze for 30 minutes.
4. Place the chocolate in the microwave until melted (30-60 seconds).
5. Dip the truffles into the melted chocolate with a skewer and place back on the baking tin. Refrigerate until ready to devour!

Strawberry Ice Cream

Serving Yields: 5
Nutritional Counts: Net Carbs: 2 g| Fat: 13 g

Ingredients:
- Strawberries – 1 cup
- Water – 1 cup
- Full-fat coconut milk – 1 can
- Glucomannan powder – 1 tsp.
- Vanilla extract – 1 tsp.
- Stevia drops – as desired

Preparation Method:
1. Using the stovetop (low heat), combine the glucomannan powder and water. Stir until it forms a gel.
2. Combine all of the fixings in a blender and mix until smooth.
3. Chill for one hour and transfer to an ice cream maker.
4. Enjoy this dessert on a hot summer day!

Smoothies for Almost Any Occasion

Avocado Raspberry Smoothie

Serving Yields: 2
Nutritional Counts: Net Carbs: 12.8 g | Fat: 20 g

Ingredients:
- Lemon juice – 3 tbsp.
- Ripened avocado - 1
- Frozen unsweetened raspberries/or your favorite - .5 cup
- Water – 1.33 cups
- Sugar equivalent – your favorite keto choice - 1 tbsp. (+) 1 tsp.

Preparation Method:
1. Combine each of the fixings in a blender until smooth.
2. Pour into chilled glasses.

Banana Bread and Blueberry Smoothie

Serving Yields: 2
Nutritional Counts: Net Carbs: 4.66 g| Fat: 23.31 g

Ingredients:
- Chia seeds – 1 tbsp.
- Golden flaxseed meal – 3 tbsp.
- Vanilla unsweetened coconut milk – from a carton – 2 cups
- Blueberries - .25 cups
- Liquid stevia – 10 drops
- MCT oil – 2 tbsp.
- Xanthan gum - .25 tsp
- Banana extract – 1.5 tsp.

Preparation Method:
1. Toss all of the fixings into a high-speed blender.
2. Give the chia seeds and flax a few minutes to absorb the moisture.
3. Blend for 1-2 minutes until everything is fully incorporated.
4. Serve in a couple of chilled glasses.

Berry Smoothie Bowl

Serving Yields: 1
Nutrition Counts: Net Carbs: 12.83 g| Fat: 54.87 g

Ingredients:
- Cooked beets - .25 cup
- Raspberries - .25 cup
- Protein powder – 1 scoop
- Hemp seeds – 1 tbsp.

Preparation Method:
1. Add everything into a bowl.
2. Mix well and enjoy.

Black Currant and Strawberry Smoothie

Serving Yields: 1
Nutritional Counts: Net Carbs: 8.7 g| Fat: 17.3 g

Ingredients:
- Chia seeds – 2 tbsp.
- Vanilla bean - .5 of 1
- Water - .5 cup
- Fresh black currants - .5 cup
- Fresh strawberries - .25 cup
- Coconut milk - .25 cup

Preparation Method:
1. Using a blender, add all of the fixings and blend until smooth.
2. Serve in a chilled glass.

Blueberry Sensation

Serving Yields: 1
Nutritional Counts: Net Carbs: 3 g | Fats: 21 g

Ingredients:
- Blueberries - .25 cup
- Coconut milk – 1 cup
- Whey protein powder – optional – 1 scoop
- Vanilla Essence – 1 tsp.
- MCT Oil – 1 tsp.

Preparation Method:
1. For a quick burst of energy, add all of the fixings into a blender.
2. Puree until it reaches the desired consistency. Add some ice if you wish.

Chocolate and Mint Smoothie

Serving Yields: 1
Nutritional Counts: Net Carbs: 6.5 g | Fats: 40.3 g

Ingredients:
- Medium avocado - .5 of 1
- Coconut milk - .25 cup
- Unsweetened cashew/almond milk – 1 cup
- Swerve/erythritol – 2 tbsp.
- Cocoa powder – 1 tbsp.
- Several fresh mint leaves
- MCT oil – 1 tbsp.
- Ice cubes - 3
- Coconut milk/whipped cream - optional

Preparation Method:
1. Mix all of the ingredients in your blender.
2. Add ice cubes as many as you like. Add the topping if desired.
3. Serve and enjoy!

Chocolate Smoothie

Serving Yields: 1 Large
Nutritional Counts: Net Carbs: 4.4 g | Fat: 46 g

Ingredients:
- Chia seeds 1-2 tbsp.
- Almond or coconut butter - 1-2 tbsp.
- Egg substitute to replace 2 large eggs
- Coconut milk/heavy whipping cream - .25 cup
- Plain/chocolate whey protein - .25 cup
- Stevia extract - 3-5 drops
- Extra-virgin coconut oil - 1 tbsp.
- Unsweetened cacao powder - 1 tbsp.
- Water - .25 cup
- Ice - .5 cup
- Vanilla extract/cinnamon - .5 tsp.

Preparation Method:
1. Combine all of the fixings into the blender.
2. Pulse until frothy. Add to a chilled glass and enjoy anytime.

Cinnamon Chocolate Smoothie

Serving Yields: 1
Nutritional Counts: Net Carbs: 4 g| Fat: 30 g

Ingredients:
- Ripened avocado - .5 of 1
- Coconut milk - .75 cup
- Cinnamon powder – 1 tsp.
- Vanilla extract - .25 tsp.
- Unsweetened cocoa powder – 2 tsp.
- Stevia – as desired
- Optional: Coconut oil – 1 tsp. or MCT oil - .5 tsp.
- Ice – 1 cup

Preparation Method:
1. Mix all of the fixings in a blender. Lastly, empty the ice.
2. Blend on the high setting for 30 seconds until thickened or until thickened.

Cinnamon Roll Smoothie

Serving Yields: 1
Nutritional Counts: Net Carbs: 0.6 g | Fats: 3.25 g

Ingredients:
- Vanilla protein powder – 2 tbsp.
- Flax meal – 1 tsp.
- Almond milk – 1 cup
- Vanilla extract - .25 tsp.
- Sweetener – 4 tsp.
- Cinnamon - .5 tsp.
- Ice – 1 cup

Preparation Method:
3. Mix all of the fixings in a blender. Lastly, empty the ice.
4. Blend on the high setting for 30 seconds until thickened or until thickened.

Easter Time Smoothie

Serving Yields: 1
Nutritional Counts: Net Carbs: 10.8 g| Fat: 23.3 g

Ingredients:
- Cantaloupe or honeydew - 1 small wedge or 1.8 oz. total
- Coconut milk/full-fat cream - .25 cup
- Avocado – 1.8 oz. - average sized
- Psyllium/chia seeds – 1 tbsp.
- Kiwifruit/berries - .25 cup
- Plain or vanilla whey protein - .25 cup
- Liquid stevia extract – 2-6 drops
- Water - .5 cup
- Ice chunks if desired – 2-3

Preparation Method:
1. Cut the avocado in half and scoop out the insides; add it to a blender.
2. Toss in the kiwi, peeled melon, and the remainder of the goodies.
3. Blend well and enjoy!

Green Choco Smoothies

Serving Yields: 2
Nutritional Counts: Net Carbs: 5.8 g| Fat: 16.3 g

Ingredients:
- Coconut cream – 1 cup
- Frozen berries - .5 cup
- Cocoa powder - .25 cup
- Granulated sweetener – 1 tbsp.

Preparation Method:
1. Use a high-speed blender to combine all of the fixings.
2. Blend until you have reached the desired consistency.
3. Serve in a couple of chilled glasses.

Maca Almond Smoothie

Serving Yields: 1
Nutritional Counts: Net Carbs: 6.2 g| Fat: 43.8 g

Ingredients:
- Unsweetened almond milk - .75 cup
- Coconut milk - .25 cup
- Unsweetened almond butter – 1 tbsp.
- Collagen powder – 1 tbsp.
- Extra-Virgin olive oil – 1 tbsp.
- Maca powder – 2 tsp.

Preparation Method:
1. Combine all of the fixings in a blender.
2. Mix well until smooth and serve in a chilled mug.

Minty Avocado and Spinach Smoothie

Serving Yields: 1
Nutritional Counts: Net Carbs: 3.6 g| Fat: 13.3 g

Ingredients:
- Fresh spinach – 1 cup
- Unsweetened almond milk - .5 cup
- Avocado - .5 of 1
- Whey protein powder – 1 scoop
- Stevia – 10 drops
- Peppermint extract - .25 tsp.
- Ice – 1 cup

Preparation Method:
1. Combine the milk, spinach, avocado, stevia, whey powder, extract, and ice in a blender.
2. Mix well until creamy, just the way you like it!

Pumpkin and Avocado Smoothie

Serving Yields: 1
Nutritional Counts: Net Carbs: 11.3 g| Fat: 69.8 g

Ingredients:
- Pumpkin puree – 3 tbsp.
- Coconut milk - full-fat - .75 cup
- MCT oil – 1 tbsp.
- Freshly chopped avocado - .5 of 1
- Pumpkin spice - .5 tsp.
- Vanilla – alcohol-free – 1 tsp.

Preparation Method:
1. Add all of the fixings to a blender.
2. Mix well until creamy smooth.
3. *Special Tip*: Not only will you enjoy the vibrant color, but the pumpkin also converts any ingested beta-carotene into vitamin A. This is a plus to help reduce the risk of some cancers, heart disease, and asthma.

Spinach and Cucumber Smoothie

Serving Yields: 1
Nutritional Counts: Net Carbs: 2.91 g| Fat: 32.34 g

Ingredients:
- Cucumber – 2.5 oz.
- Spinach –2 handfuls.
- Coconut milk – from a carton – 1 cup
- Cubes of ice – 7 Large
- Liquid stevia – 12 drops
- MCT Oil – 1-2 tbsp.
- Xanthan gum - .25 tsp.

Preparation Method:
1. Peel and cube the cucumber. Combine all of the fixings in a high-speed blender (ex. Ninja).
2. Blend for 1-2 minutes until it's creamy like you like it.
3. Pour into a chilled glass and enjoy the healthy drink anytime!

Cold Beverages

Green Coffee Shake

Serving Yields: 4
Nutritional Counts: Net Carbs: 4.4 g| Fat: 24.9 g

Ingredients:
- Full-fat coconut milk - 1 can - 13.5 fl. oz.
- Chilled brewed coffee (decaf or regular – 1.5 cup
- Unsweetened almond butter – 2 tbsp.
- Genuine Health vegan greens - vanilla-flavored – 1 tbsp.
- For Serving: Ice cubes - 8

Preparation Method:
1. Combine all of the fixings except for the ice in the blender jug.
2. Pulse until smooth or about 10 seconds.
3. Portion into your chosen glasses and add the ice cubes.
4. Serve and smile!

Iced Blended Coffee

Serving Yields: 1
Nutritional Counts: Net Carbs: 64.7 g| Fat: 99.3 g

Ingredients:
- Hemp hearts – 2 tbsp. or 1 tbsp. almond butter
- Brewed coffee/favorite tea – 1.75 cups
- Cacao butter -10 g. – 4-5 wafers
- Alcohol-free stevia – 4 drops
- Coconut- 1 tbsp. or MCT oil
- Ground cinnamon - .25 tsp.
- Ground vanilla bean - .25 tsp
- Cubes of ice – 4-6

Ingredients for the topping:
- Cacao nibs – 1 tsp.
- Coconut whipped cream - .25 cup

Preparation Method:
1. Measure out all of the fixings and add to a blender; mix until creamy smooth.
2. Toss in the ice and continue until it's the way you like it.
3. Serve with the chosen toppings.

McKeto Strawberry Milkshake

Serving Yields: 1
Nutritional Counts: Net Carbs: 2.42 g| Fat: 38.85

Ingredients:
- Heavy cream - .25 cup
- Coconut milk – from a carton - .75 cup
- Sugar-free Strawberry Torani Syrup – 2 tbsp.
- Xanthan gum - .25 tsp.
- MCT oil – 1 tbsp.
- Cubes of ice - 7

Preparation Method:
1. Combine all of the fixings in a blender. (such as Ninja).
2. Combine for 1-2 minutes until it's like you enjoy it.
3. Serve in a chilled glass.

Hot Beverages

Coconut – Coffee Mug

Serving Yields: 1
Nutritional Counts: Net Carbs: 2 g| Fat: 27 g

Ingredients:
- Coconut oil – 1 tbsp.
- Ground flaxseeds – 2 tbsp.
- Coconut flakes – unsweetened – 2 tbsp.
- Liquid sweetener – as desired
- Unsweetened black coffee - .5 cup

Preparation Method:
1. Combine the flaxseeds, coconut oil, and coconut flakes in a mug.
2. Pour in the prepared coffee. Add the sweetener of choice and enjoy.

Creamy Hot Cocoa in the Crockpot

Serving Yields: 4
Nutritional Counts: Net Carbs: 3 g| Fat: 5 g

Ingredients:
- Unsweetened almond milk – 3 cups
- Salt - .25 tsp.
- Stevia – 8-10 packets
- Vanilla – 1 tsp.
- Half and Half - .25 cup
- Cocoa powder – unsweetened - .25 cup (+) 2 tbsp.

Preparation Method:
1. Combine all of the fixings in the crockpot.
2. Set the timer for two hours using the low setting (covered).
3. Stir occasionally. Serve in a warm mug and enjoy!

Energizing Latte

Serving Yields: 1
Nutritional Counts: Net Carbs: -0- g| Fat: 25.8 g

Ingredients:
- Stevia – 1 drop
- Brewed coffee – 8 oz.
- Cacao butter - 1 tbsp.
- Hemp hearts - 1 tbsp.
- MCT oil - 1 tbsp.
- Grass-fed collagen - 1 tbsp.

Preparation Method:
1. First, brew the coffee and combine all of the fixings in a blender (omit the collagen).
2. Mix for 1 minute and add the collagen (the last 10 sec.).
3. Enjoy before you start your hectic day.

A Final Word

You now have a ton of recipes to choose from as a vegan. Before you begin, it is advisable to visit your doctor. If you are attempting to lose weight using the ketogenic diet techniques, you need to be aware of some possible medications that can contribute to weight gain. Do you take any of these?

- Oral contraceptives
- Anti-Depressants
- Epilepsy drugs
- Blood pressure medications
- Allergy medicines
- Antibiotics

As you begin your dieting using your keto lifestyle changes, you will notice some obvious differences. Here are some examples:

Keto Flu
The diet can make you a bit confused, irritable, nauseous, cause you to have diarrhea or constipation, muscle cramping, bloated, and lethargic. You may also suffer from a lingering headache. Sugar cravings and heart palpations may also be present. Just like the traditional flu, the keto flu may have a total run of 24-72-hours. Several days into the plan should remedy these issues. If not, just add 1/2 teaspoon of salt to a glass of water. Drink it to help ease the side effects. It might be necessary to do this once a day for about the first week.

Note: It could take about 15-20 minutes before it helps.

Intense urine odor

The color change is due to your body adjusting and entering ketosis.

Adjustments in the digestive system
As your body is challenged by additional fiber and other foods, you may experience bouts of constipation or diarrhea. Water also helps with dehydration but may also cause intestinal issues. Try reducing new foods until the transitional phase of ketosis is concluded; it should clear up with time. You may also be lacking beneficial bacteria. Try consuming fermented foods to increase your probiotics and aid digestion. You can also benefit from Vitamin B, omega-3 fatty acids, and beneficial enzymes. Take a dose of Milk of Magnesia if other suggestions don't work for you.

Heart palpitations
It is possible you will have heart palpitations as a result of insufficient intake of salt or dehydration. Adjust your menu plan with a few more carbs to see if they subside. If you don't begin to feel better soon, you should seek emergency care.

Changes in sleeping pattern
If you have been asleep for over eight hours, that good night of sleep will throw your body into ketosis. If you are new to the low-carb and high-fat diet plan, it will take time to achieve optimal fat-burning status. Your body has depended on bringing in carbs and glucose; it will not readily give up carbs and start to crave saturated fats. Insomnia is a normal side effect.

Vitamin supplements can sometimes remedy the problem that can be caused by a lowered insulin and serotonin level. For a quick fix, try one-half of a tablespoon of fruit spread and a square of chocolate. It really does work! However, you still need to count the carbs (if any) of your homemade remedy.

Don't eat dinner when it's close to bedtime. You should consume the last meal of the day approximately two to three hours before it's time to retire for the day. If you're prone to Gastroesophageal Reflux Disease or GERD, eating before bed is also a sure-fire way of making the matter worse, even a snack will cause issues. Try half of an egg, cherry tomatoes, or a few almonds if you cannot make it to the next meal.

Insomnia
If you have problems sleeping a full eight hours, then you are like about 75% of Americans. According to the Centers for Disease Control and Prevention (CDC), that equals to about one out of three people who could have issues with type 2

diabetes, cardiovascular disease, obesity, or high blood pressure/hypertension because of the lack of sleep.

Therefore, the less sleep you get, the harder it is to drop those extra pounds. According to another study, individuals who slept just four hours experienced a 24% jump in calorie intake, increased hunger drive, decreased leptin levels (the appetite control hormone), and increased ghrelin levels (the appetite hormone that triggers hunger).

You tend to snack more and add up those calories quickly without the right amount of restful sleep. These are a few of the elements that could be causing your sleepless nights:

- Substance or alcohol abuse
- Certain illnesses
- Depression, anxiety, and stress
- Hormonal conditions and changes
- Sleep apnea
- Certain medications
- Stimulants, including too much caffeine

If you have insomnia and cannot sleep, have a **serving of Spiced Hot Toddy** for zero carbs; it only takes about ten minutes.

Spiced Hot Toddy

Nutrition Facts: 110 Calories
   Note: You have -0- g Protein, Total Fats, and Net Carbs

What You Need:

- Bourbon – 1.5 oz.
- Boiling water – 2 oz.
- Fresh lemon juice - .25 of 1
- Whole cloves – 2
- Sweetener of choice – to taste
- Cinnamon stick – 1
- Garnish with a dash of ground nutmeg

How to Prepare:
1. Combine all of the liquid components in a small pot on the stovetop.
2. Lower the heat and add the spices and cinnamon stick. Simmer for about 3 minutes. Sprinkle with a dusting of nutmeg.
3. When ready, just pour into a mug to kick your worst cold (or anything else).
4. You can make multiple servings in a crockpot if you want to serve the crowd. Just keep the lid on the cooker.
5. Note: Just remember, this is not an open invitation to drink alcohol; it is just one option to consider.

Risks for those with diabetes

If you are diabetic and want to begin a ketogenic diet plan, there are a few things you need to keep in mind. The keto diet has proven benefits for individuals who have type 2 diabetes, but you should be a bit more cautious if you have type 1 diabetes. There is not as much research at this time on other forms of diabetes.

Keep in mind that it's the quality, not the quantity, of the carbs you consume since you do not want to slice them from your diet plan entirely. Have a talk with your doctor to help you make a healthy choice for your needs.

Don't cut out the carbs too quickly. According to Prevention, it isn't wise to dramatically cut carbs from your diet, especially if you are taking insulin or oral diabetes medications. This could result in low blood glucose (hypoglycemia). You want to lower the carb intake gradually.

Don't consume too many carbs either. You need to be sure you follow a strict carb count guideline since you don't realize how many points each food has and how quickly they add up. In addition to other side effects, you will also have bouts of constipation, keto flu, or possible dehydration. However, these are just small bumps in the road for most individuals.

Be aware of diabetic ketoacidosis. According to Mayo Clinic, when diabetics produce high levels of ketones, it can potentially become a severe complication. This triggers when your body does not receive an appropriate amount of insulin, which converts the sugar into energy. Therefore, if it goes into "starvation mode," it will break down the fuel at an alarmingly fast rate. Don't take the chance; stay in touch with your doctor for the best results using the ketogenic way of living.

Keep Your Final Goals in Mind While on the Keto Journey

It is a long trip to keep and maintain ketosis. This segment is a reminder of the essential elements for you to have a smooth transition to ketosis and beyond.

Expect plateaus with your weight loss plan
If you have ever dieted before, you already know you will reach spans of time where your weight loss will reach a level out.

That's merely a segment of weight loss that can't be moderated. All you need to do is remain consistent; the weight loss will return.

Practice mindful eating
It is vital to take a few extra moments to enjoy the flavors and textures of your food. The ketogenic diet will provide all of the nourishment to remain successful dieting. **Enjoy your time with the conversation of a friend or family member. Drink your water and sip your tea or coffee. Feel satisfied and enjoy the moment; stop rushing around at dinner time.**

Limit psychological and physical stress during evening hours
It is essential for you to recharge and take the evening hours to relax to improve your sleep hygiene. Try to leave work – at work; deal with the issues in the morning. If you are going through a tough time or working long hours, you tend to forget items you may "munch" on as you are working. Make it a point to write down everything you eat.

Working long hours can be beneficial for knocking off those pounds. However, it can also cause you to be restless and can lead to post-workout insomnia if you have done strenuous physical activities on your evenings off. No matter what the case, slow down for at least an hour or more before attempting to retire for the evening.

Limit your screen time and dim the lights
Your production of melatonin has a negative impact if the blue screen lights are left on your computer, tablets, or cell phone. Shut it all down about an hour before bedtime. You might not be able to shut the phone down completely, but use an app

that will lower the lighting. The thought of missing a call can keep your mind wired at alert, which will make sleep more difficult. In short, limit your exposure to the blue lights.

Reassess and adjust your goals as needed
After you have adjusted your body to the ketogenic dieting plan, you can start using an intermittent fasting method if you choose to take that route. Be willing to change your goals as you make progress. By starting small, you leave the door open so you can make more significant challenges as you proceed through the plan.

Always remain honest with yourself
Even though ketogenic foods will provide you with essential vitamins and nutrients without a lot of junk foods, it doesn't necessarily mean that it is automatically the right option for your needs.

Think about how disciplined you are, what your relationship with food is like, and how healthy you are in general. It is a lot easier to be realistic about your chance of success and decide to look elsewhere before you get started in earnest than after struggling with and failing after a week or more of serious effort. With Keto, you will be satisfied and less likely to fail versus other dieting methods. You have many choices to succeed in your weight loss regimen.

Take a break
When starting out, it is essential to understand that the transition period can be somewhat tricky, and it will be worse for some. As such, it is a good idea to choose a time to start the transition that is relatively free from stress or otherwise hectic plans. You are likely going to have a hard time making the

change. Anything else on your plate is probably going to take a hit. "Forewarned is forearmed," however, and planning for the development will make it easier to manage.

Reward yourself
Especially when you are first starting out, it is important to reward a successful week on your new way of eating with some type of splurge. As long as you don't let it get out of hand, there is no harm in having an extra decadent dessert; just make sure it remains in the keto carb levels. Better yet, go on a new adventure with the family.

More about those plateaus
Okay, you have made it this far, and you realize there will be bumps in the road during your time headed toward ketosis. These are a few that others have made, so you can dodge them. This is always a good review time!

Plateau 1: Not tracking your carbs properly
As you enter into ketosis, your hunger generation is generally improved. Since ketogenic foods can be calorically-dense, you need to be sure that you are tracking and weighing all of your food. That's the only way you will maintain a deficit.

Plateau 2: Not eating the right veggie and fruit choices
It's pretty simple to avoid this issue with a side of broccoli or cauliflower. You can also have a healthy side salad here or some of the delicious fruits provided in your previous chapters.

Plateau 3: Not having an actual deficit

Once you have lost an adequate amount of weight, it might be essential to reassess your macros. Since you weigh much less, you will also need to lower your food consumption.

Plateau 4: Snacking mindlessly
Make sure you are genuinely hungry before you decide to splurge. Have a large glass of water. You have to be mindful since snacking can be caused by negative emotions or just plain boredom. Food is for fuel to run your body. Therefore, eating when you aren't hungry might distort your body's natural cues. After all, hunger is a part of the weight loss equation. Your body likes the balance and wants to hold onto its current weight. That is why, on some days, you may be hungrier than others. Power through those weak moments or enjoy a healthy snack.

Plateau 5: Watch out for hidden carbs
Remember, the ideal carb consumption is at or below 20-25 net carbs while using the keto plan – especially when you begin your diet plan. Be sure you are tracking the carbs and not eating too many foods that might have carbohydrates lurking. As an example, tofu can have different carbs depending on the brand. Always check your labels when shopping for your keto needs.

Benefits of Ketogenic Diet as a Vegan

Seizure reduction for epilepsy patients
Reductions in seizures have occurred in children who have successfully used the ketogenic diet. The therapeutic keto diet used for epilepsy often restricts the carbs to fewer than 15 grams of carbs daily to further drive up the ketone levels.

Don't try to reach these levels unless you have the supervision of a medical professional.

Accelerated fat loss for overweight and obese individuals
Many people exceed what is considered healthy figures when it comes to weight. It is imperative to use the keto diet plan to get started on the right path for weight loss.

Prediabetes and diabetes improvements
With the excess fat removed using the keto plan, you will also have noted improvement of pre-diabetes, type-2 diabetes, and metabolic syndrome.

Joint pain and stiffness is significantly improved
Grain-based foods are abolished from your diet using the keto plan. It's believed the grains can be one of the biggest causes of pain or chronic illness.

Improved thinking skills
You might become confused as you consume high-fat foods since your brain is approximately 60% fat by weight. It can maintain itself and work at full capacity using ketosis.

Cancer patient relief
Several types of cancer and slow tumor growths are being treated by using the keto diet technique.

A slowed process of those with Alzheimer's disease
The disease's progression can be delayed and the symptoms reduced with the keto plan.

Lower blood pressures
It is wise to speak with your doctor about lowering your medications while on the plan. If you begin to feel dizzy, this is an indication that the lack of carbs is working.

Cholesterol profile improvement
An arterial buildup is typically associated with triglyceride and cholesterol levels, which have been proven to improve with the keto diet plan.

Repaired gum disease and tooth decay issues
The pH balance in your mouth is influenced by sugar intake. The plan should help your gum issues subside after about three months.

Conclusion

I hope each segment of the Vegan Keto Cookbook was informative and able to provide you with all the tools you need to achieve whatever your goals may be. If you are searching for a well-rounded diet for your child, these tips could be useful for training the way of a vegan diet:

- Let the children help.
- Start the process with foods the child already likes.
- Provide a packed lunch, so you would know your child has the right types of foods.
- Mix up the menu and keep it interesting.
- Plan meals in advance.

Keep it simple for children; try some of these great finger foods:
- Pear slices
- Apple slices
- Banana
- Avocado
- Sweet potato cubes and slices
- Carrot sticks and rounds

Keep track of which foods are best liked by your child. Always keep a watch while you provide the crunchy snacks. Some of these foods will require adult supervision. As with any diet, you may have side effects. The ketogenic plan offers several ways to remedy the issues.

The next step is to decide which deliciously healthy meal you want to try first and prepare a list of each of the ingredients you need. It is also advisable to make a list of staples which will be used with many of the vegan type recipes. You can use the information provided within to prepare tasty dishes that your family and friends will rave about for quite some time. You have the total fats and net carbs calculated by Keto standards, so have fun!

Finally, if you found *"The Vegan Keto Cookbook 2021: Over 190 High-Fat Low-Carb Plant-Based Recipes to Shed and Heal You from the Inside Out"* useful in any way, a review is always appreciated!

Index for the Recipes

Chapter 1: Morning and Brunch Specialties 27
    Bulletproof Coffee 27
    Bulletproof Tea 29

Pancake Time 30
    Cinnamon Roll Pancakes 30
    Coconut Pancakes 32
    Crispy Flaxseed Waffles 33
    Flaxseed Pancakes 35
    Scallion Pancakes 36

Other Delicious Choices 38
    Almonds and Chips Breakfast Cereal 38
    Avocado – Carrot and Tahini Breakfast Bowl 39
    Bagel Thins for Breakfast 40
    Berry and Nut Cereal 42
    Blueberry Breakfast Cake – Flourless and Gluten-Free 43
    Bran Muffins – Gluten-Free 45
    Breakfast Quiche 47
    Cinnamon Roll Muffins 48
    Macadamia Breakfast Bars 50
    Maple Walnut Breakfast Cereal 51
    Minty Eggplant Hash Browns 52
    Muesli in the Raw 53
    Peanut Butter Breakfast Cereal 54
    Psyllium Breakfast Mix 55
    Pumpkin Pie Breakfast Cereal 56
    Scrambled Tofu 57
    Seed and Nut-Packed Bread 58
    Vanilla and Turmeric Breakfast Cereal 60

Oatmeal and Porridge Favorites 61
    Berries and Hemp Seeds 61
    Blueberry Porridge 62
    Fudge Oatmeal 64

Overnight Oat Options 65
    Alternative #1: Vanilla Oats: The Base 65
    Alternative #2: Pumpkin Spice Latte Overnight Oats 66
    Alternative #3: Fudge Overnight Oats 67

Porridge Options 68
    Delicious Plain Porridge 68
    Porridge with Cinnamon and Hemp Hearts 69

Chapter 2: Delicious Meals and Salads 70

Meals 70
    Asparagus and Mushrooms with Cauliflower Risotto 70
    Asparagus and Tofu Stir Fry 73
    Broccoli Noodles and Tofu 75
    Cauliflower Tabbouleh 77
    Collard Green Wraps 78
    Crispy Tofu and Cauliflower Rice 79
    Eggplant Lasagna 81
    Falafel with Tahini Sauce 83
    French Style Ratatouille 85
    Green Panini 87
    Sesame Tofu and Eggplant 88

Salads 90
    Arugula and Blueberry Salad 90
    Asian Zucchini Salad 91
    Asparagus and Artichoke Salad 92
    Avocado and Greens Salad 93
    Avocado Papaya Salad 94
    Bell Pepper and Asparagus Salad 95
    Caesar Vegan Salad 96
    Courgette Salad and Herbed Vinaigrette 97
    Eggplant Salad 98
    Kale Salad and Blueberry Dressing 99
    Lemony Brussel Sprout Salad 101
    Pear and Dates with Special Cider Dressing 102
    Pecan Cauliflower Salad 103
    Simple Green Salad with Lemon Vinaigrette 104
    Sun-Dried Tomato Salad and Cider Dressing 106

Thai Peanut Zucchini Noodle Salad 107

Chapter 3: Healthy Soups – Stews and Chowder 109

Beetroot Ginger Soup 109
Broccoli and Cauliflower Soup 111
Cabbage and Beet Soup 112
Chili – Vegan Style 113
Chilled Minty Avocado Soup 114
Creamy Avocado Soup 115
Creamy Red Gazpacho Soup 116
Creamy Tomato Soup 118
Ginger Cauliflower Stew 120
Mushroom Soup 121
Red Onion Soup 123
Spanish Soup 124
Spinach and Turnip Soup 125
Superfood Keto Soup 126
Thai Pumpkin Soup 128
Turmeric Cabbage Soup 130
Zucchini Basil Soup 131

Chapter 4: Vegan Creams - Sauces and Dips 132

Avocado Mayo 132
Barbecue Sauce 133
Coconut Whipped Cream 134
Eggplant Bruschetta 135
Guacamole 136
Hummus and Avocado 137
Ketchup 138
Lemon and Jalapeno Cream Sauce 139
Mayo – Vegan Style 140
Nutella Spread 141
Peanut Sauce 142
Portobello Mushroom Bruschetta 143
Slow-Cooked Summer Bruschetta 144
Spinach Avocado Dip 145
Tahini and Cilantro Sauce 147
Tofu or Seitan Marinades 148

Vegan Sour Cream 151
Veggie Salsa 152

Chapter 5: Appetizers – Sides and Snacks 153

Sides 153

Basil Zoodles and Olives 153
Beetroot and Pesto Noodles 154
Brussels Sprouts and Cashew Dip 155
Cabbage Slaw 156
Carrot and Zucchini Noodles in Thai Sauce 157
Cauliflower and Artichoke Couscous 158
Cauliflower Bites with Ranch Dip 159
Cherry Tomatoes and Zucchini Pasta 160
Chili and Coconut Cauliflower Rice 161
Coconut Cauliflower Rice 162
Creamy Curry Low-Carb Noodle Bowl 163
Edamame Kelp Noodles 165
Garlicky Mushrooms 166
Grilled Eggplant and Zucchini 167
Indian Curried Cauliflower 168
Kelp Noodles with Peanut Butter Sauce 169
Lime and Chili Carrot Noodles 170
Mediterranean Spaghetti Squash 171
Mushroom, Broccoli, and Squash Noodles 173
Nutty Pesto Zucchini 174
Pesto Kelp Noodles 175
Roasted Beetroot Noodles 176
Roasted Broccoli 177
Roasted Green Cabbage 179
Roasted Kale and Squash 180
Spaghetti Squash 181
Sriracha Grilled Asparagus 182
Teriyaki Grilled Eggplant 183
Tofu Pizza Sticks 184
Turnip Fries 185
Turnip and Courgette Hash Browns 186
Zucchini Noodles and Avocado Sauce 187

Snack Time Treats 188

Carrot Cake Bites 188
Chocolate Granola 189
Chocolate Protein Bars 190
Cinnamon Granola 191
Coconut and Peanut Butter Balls 192
Fudge Balls 193
Loaded Nut-Packed Coconut Granola 194
Mushroom Chips 196
Pecan and Maple Fat Bars 197
Peanut Butter Fat Bombs 198
Peanut Tofu Wrap 199
Roasted Radish Chips 200
Sweet Potato Toast 201
Zucchini Chips 202

Chapter 6: Desserts – Smoothies and Beverages 203

Pudding Specialties 203
Avocado and Chocolate Pudding 203
Chia Chocolate Pudding 205
Chia Raspberry Pudding 207
Chia Strawberry Pudding 208
Coconut Chia and Turmeric Pudding 209
Pumpkin and Peanut Butter Pudding 210

Other Delicious Desserts 211
Avocado Chocolate Mousse 211
Banana Bread 213
Cashew and Blueberry Cheesecake 214
Chilled Avocado and Strawberry Bowl 215
Cinnamon and Pumpkin Fudge 216
Coconut Bombs 217
Coconut Cupcakes 218
Coconut Maple Fudge 220
Coconut and Peanut Butter Balls 221
Coconut and Strawberry Bars 222
Dairy-Free Chocolate Silk Pie 223
Lime Avocado Popsicles 225
Mexican Chocolate Avocado Ice Cream 226
Minty Berries in A Dish 228

Pecan and Blueberry Crumble 229
Pumpkin Truffles 230
Raspberry Coconut Bark 231
Raspberry Truffles 232
Strawberry Ice Cream 233

Smoothies for Almost Any Occasion 234
Avocado Raspberry Smoothie 234
Banana Bread and Blueberry Smoothie 235
Berry Smoothie Bowl 236
Black Currant and Strawberry Smoothie 237
Blueberry Sensation 238
Chocolate and Mint Smoothie 239
Chocolate Smoothie 240
Cinnamon Chocolate Smoothie 241
Cinnamon Roll Smoothie 242
Easter Time Smoothie 243
Green Choco Smoothies 244
Maca Almond Smoothie 245
Minty Avocado and Spinach Smoothie 246
Pumpkin and Avocado Smoothie 247
Spinach and Cucumber Smoothie 248

Cold Beverages 249
Green Coffee Shake 249
Iced Blended Coffee 250
McKeto Strawberry Milkshake 251

Hot Beverages 252
Coconut – Coffee Mug 252
Creamy Hot Cocoa in the Crockpot 253
Energizing Latte 254

www.ingramcontent.com/pod-product-compliance
Lightning Source LLC
Chambersburg PA
CBHW081344070526
44578CB00005B/714